Keto Diet Cookbook After 50

The Ultimate Ketogenic Diet Guide for Seniors | 28–Day Meal Plan | Lose Up To 20 Pounds In 3 Weeks

By Tiffany Diamond

Content

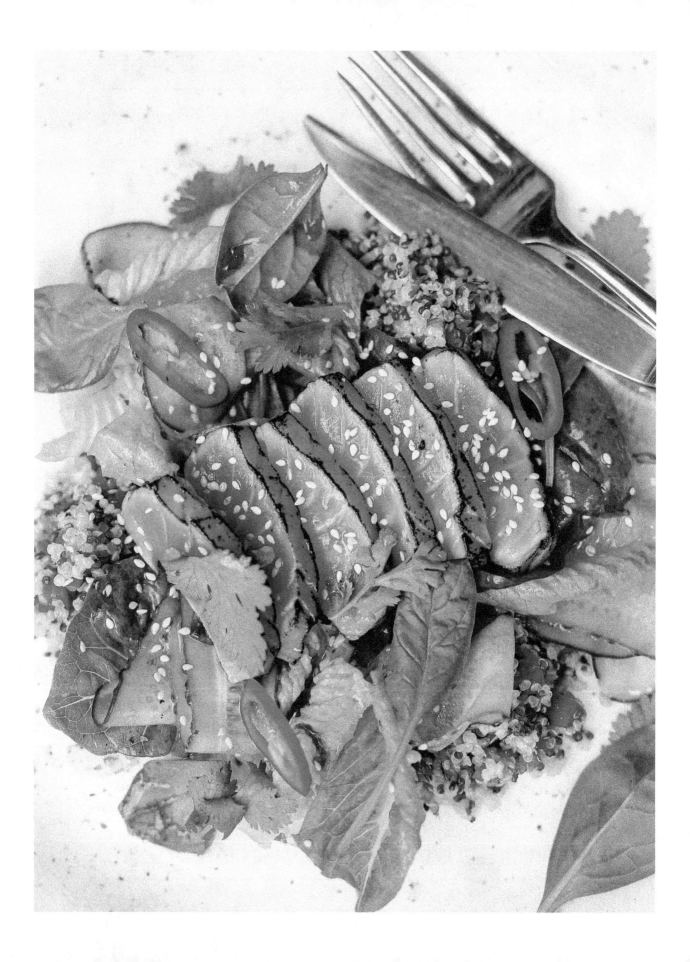

INTRODUCTION

Are you over 50 years old and looking for a weight loss solution? You can achieve this by following one of the most popular diets—the Keto diet. The Keto diet will help you burn excess fat and retrieve your youth. Also, you won't feel starved when dieting anymore. The Keto diet allows you to eat meats and fats, and you'll feel satiety with no guilt. You may wonder why the Keto diet is so magical.

First, you need to know what the Keto diet is. The Keto diet is a high-fat, low-carb, medium-protein diet. The macro nutrient breakdown is 70-90% of fat calories, 15-25% of protein calories, and 5-10% of carbohydrate calories. The fat proportion is much higher than people consume traditionally, and it is imperative to note that these fats should be mostly unsaturated fats, including polyunsaturated fat; not the bad fat, such as trans-fat. The good fats are essential because they are the key to heal your body and lose weight.

As the years go by, you will need to have essential nutrients, which can improve your immune system, brain, and eyes as well as speed up your metabolism. In this book, we will discuss what the Keto diet is, what ketosis is, and give you a deep understanding of how it all works. We will also teach you how to customize your calories according to your basic metabolic value. Besides, you will know how to adjust nutrients corresponding to the needs of your body. Age should not be a factor as far as not being able to live a better life. When you are eating the right foods with rich nutrition, your body will know this, and therefore, work better. Most of the foods in the recipes of this book can be easily found at your local store. You will also learn a lot of practical information from this book that you can apply when executing the diet.

This book will open the door of the Keto diet for you and lead you on the right path to a healthy lifestyle. What are you waiting for? Let's explore it together!

Chapter 1 The Keto Diet Basics

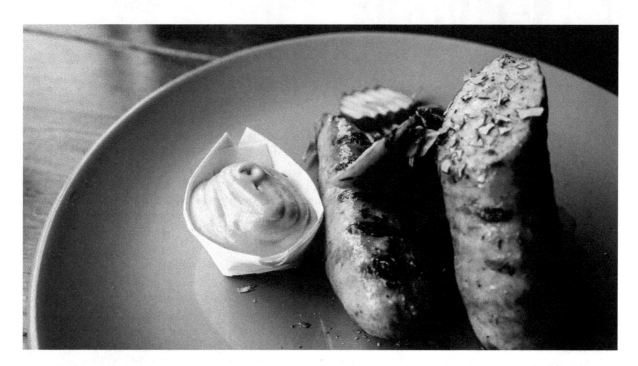

What's Keto Diet?

The Keto diet was developed in 1924 by Dr. Russel as a treatment for epileptic patients. He observed that when the body was in ketosis, it could prevent epileptic symptoms. Over time, people have applied this diet in their lives in order to enhance their quality of life. They have found that there are many benefits to sticking with this diet, including healing brain injuries, preventing a heart attack, stabilizing blood glucose levels, treating autism, etc.

The Keto diet is composed of a high amount of fat, a low amount of carbohydrates, and a medium amount of protein. Most body cells prefer to use blood sugar as fuel, which usually comes from carbohydrates. However, when the level of carbohydrates is low, the body will be forced to break down fats in order to supply energy, and then body will produce ketones as fuel. The Keto diet switches the sugar-fueled mode into a ketone-fueled mode. As the level of ketones elevates, a metabolic state called ketosis forms. The body usually starts adapting to ketosis after two weeks if taking in 20 to 50 grams of carbohydrates each day. It is important to note that the time varies depending on individuals; some people need more restriction to get into ketosis while others require a shorter time.

As mentioned above, with a high proportion of fat, the Keto diet includes fat-rich foods, such as meats, cheeses, fish, butter, oils, seeds, and nuts. Glucose is the primary source of energy for your cells in the body, and the body tends to utilize glucose for energy. When you eat too many carbs, the glucose cannot be burned completely, and it will be converted into glycogen. Glycogen will be stored in the organs and in other parts of your body, finally leading to obesity. Glucose is not the most efficient source of energy; it can bring serious health problems. Obesity, type II diabetes, heart diseases, and many diabetic problems are associated with high-carbohydrate diets.

Is The Keto Diet Healthy for People after 50?

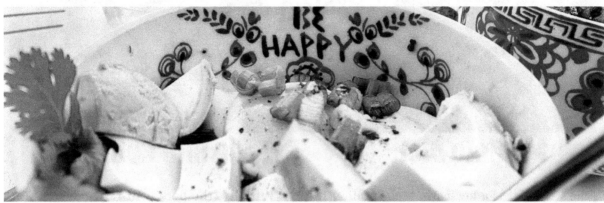

As people age, we need foods that supply us adequate energy and are easily digested As people age, we need foods that supply us with adequate energy and are easily digested in order to reduce the chances of developing lifelong diseases. The key point of the Keto diet is to utilize the fats for energy, which is a better fuel supply than that of high-carb diets. When it comes to dieting, you may feel confused and at a loss. How can you know whether the diet is right for you? This book aims to help people who are over 50 years of age make the right choice. It will help you understand various diets and select the one that suits your age best in order to revitalize your body while preventing chronic illnesses.

By following the Keto diet, you will avoid food addictions and binge or emotional eating, but choose healthier foods to feed your body; thus, feeling clear-headed and vigorous.

Research has shown solid evidence that the Keto diet can improve brain functions significantly since it plays an important role in brain neuroprotection. Your brain cells will become more active and memory loss will be improved. Some studies suggest that the Keto diet can help prevent Alzheimer's, Parkinson's, Autism, sleep disorders, etc. It can reduce insulin resistance, shape your mind, and help you keep a pleasant mood. Besides its weight loss effectiveness, many people over 50 shed stubborn fat around their waist and hips through this diet.

Even though the diet is based on fats, you should intake healthy fats as much as possible and avoid processed foods, saturated fats, and trans-fats. Eating whole foods is the first step to building a better immune system and a better mood. Choose the Keto diet and enjoy the benefits it brings!

So why is the Keto diet the most preferred type of diet for people over 50?

The body has different metabolic pathways that are essential for the production of energy; however, some are used more often than others. One of the body's preferred sources of fuel is usually glucose, and this is the simplest form of carbohydrates. Carbohydrates include simple carbs and complex carbs. Most of the flour, bread, starch, and sugar that we consume is simple carbs and can be absorbed by the body and broken down into glucose quickly. On the other hand, complex carbohydrates, such as most green-leaf vegetables, are digested slowly and the insoluble fiber can't be absorbed, which is healthier compared with simple carbohydrates.

When the glucose level in the body is low, the body will break down fat into energy, which is a better way to supply fuels to our bodies. This is the mechanism of the Keto diet in order to avoid ailments and diseases, lose weight, and heal our bodies.

The Keto diet is considered as a miracle diet because it improves your health and allows your cells to rejuvenate quickly. It also makes you feel stronger and younger. You can have all these benefits by following the diet and taking your body and health to a whole new level.

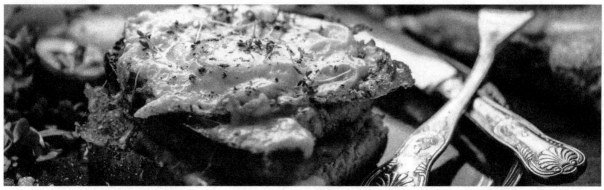

Types of Keto Diet

Getting into Ketosis

The Keto diet is a low-carb, high-fat diet. It is known to shift the body's metabolism from a carb-supply mode towards a fat-supply mode. There are many versions of the Keto diet, including:

The Standard Keto Diet

This is a very low-carb, moderate-protein, high-fat diet. It usually contains 75% fats, 20% proteins, and 5% carbohydrates.

The Cyclic Keto Diet

This diet involves adhering to a standard Keto diet for five to six days per week followed by one to two days of higher carb consumption, called "refeeding days," which are meant to replenish your body's depleted glucose reserves.

The Targeted Keto Diet

This is a diet that will allow you to add carbs when you have hard workouts.

The High Protein Keto Diet

This is similar to the standard Keto diet, but it has a high proportion of proteins. The ratio is often 60% fat, 5% carbs, and 35% proteins.

It is important to know that the favorable Keto diet for people over 50 is the standard Keto diet. Cyclic and targeted Keto diets are more advanced and are often used by athletes and bodybuilders.

Initially, the body will rely more on free fatty acids before moving on to ketones; however, cells that are unable to use free fatty acids will use ketones. The brain cannot use fatty acids because they cannot cross the blood-brain barrier. Therefore, as the glucose reserves continue to diminish, the liver will begin a myriad of processes to convert the free fatty acids into ketones. Once the glucose reserves are depleted to a certain extent, the body will enter a state of ketosis. This is a state where the body relies on ketone bodies for energy.

Ketones are composed of three chemicals: acetoacetate, acetone, and beta-hydroxybutyrate. In mild ketosis, acetoacetate is the primary ketone produced. In deeper states, beta-hydroxybutyrate becomes the major energy source.

Nutritional ketosis is defined as the situation where ketone concentration is from 0.5 mmol per liter to 3 mmol per liter. The major factor that should be considered is that when the ketone concentration rises too high (above 10 mmol per liter), it will result in ketoacidosis, which may lead to death in extreme cases. However, this only occurs among alcoholics, diabetics, and people undergoing starvation.

Once you are in a state of ketosis, the body will excrete small amounts of ketones in your urine and breath. The liver cannot use ketones for energy, although it can process it into pyruvate, and the brain cannot use ketone bodies at all. Therefore, the system will be forced to generate glucose through gluconeogenesis, and even in a deep state of ketosis, the body will still produce some glucose.

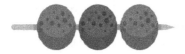

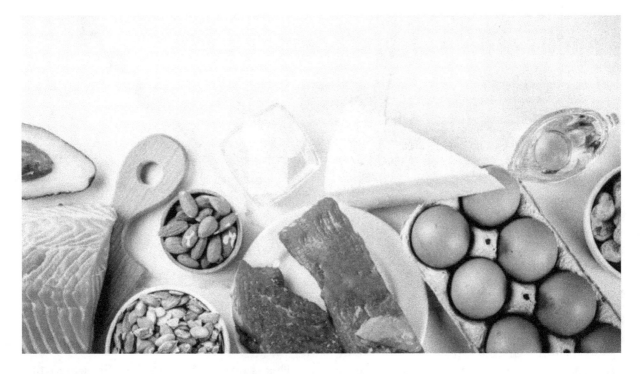

How to Know You Are In Ketosis

Keto-adaptation is a process in which the body will adapt to ketones as a source of energy instead of glucose. After you get into ketosis, the body ramps up the metabolic pathways in order to produce ketones; therefore, you will not lack the energy to run vital organs. The body will produce ketones immediately when the glucose level reduces to a certain threshold. The process of keto-adaptation will take two to four weeks. During this time, you will experience symptoms similar to a sugar rush or a mild head flu, which is called keto flu.

One of the useful ways of testing whether or not you are in ketosis is by using ketone test strips. They will let you know the level of ketones in your body. Another way is by using a blood glucose monitor. However, you do not have to go to complex measures or expensive ways to know if you are in ketosis. Symptoms or indicators that will let you know that you have gotten into ketosis include:

Increased Urination
Keto is a natural diuretic, and you will find yourself going to the bathroom more often than before. You will also drink a great amount of water.

Dry Mouth
The more fluids you excrete, the more likely you will experience dry mouth. This is normal because it's just a signal that your body is telling you that you need more electrolytes.

Dragon Breath
Acetone, a ketone, is excreted through urine and breath and your breath will smell like nail polish. Having dragon breath means that you have gotten into ketosis.

Reduced Hunger And Increased Energy
This is the most obvious sign of ketosis. You will find that you will not feel as hungry as often and you can go longer without food.

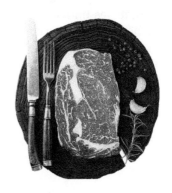

Benefits of Keto Diet for People after 50

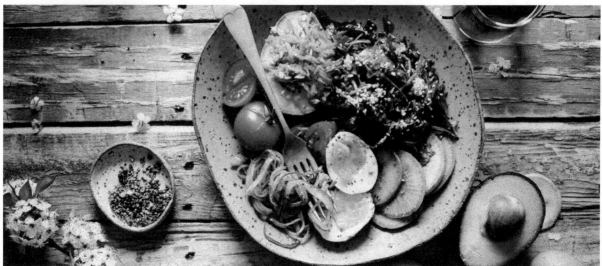

The essence of the Keto diet cannot be emphasized further because the process usually results in a myriad of changes that are beneficial to the body. When you are on the Keto diet, you will experience new aspects in your life, and the cell rejuvenation process will begin at a rapid rate. Here are some benefits of the Keto diet for people over 50.

Fat Loss Without Hunger

Weight loss experts recommend the Keto diet because it is highly effective in executing long-term weight loss. In essence, you will have better glycemic index control, and you can lose more fat within a shorter period of time than with other diets. The Keto diet is known to reduce your appetite and you will not feel hungry as often as you did, consequently not consuming unnecessary calories.

Blood Sugar Control

One of the main problems that people suffering from diabetes undergo is the inability of their body to handle insulin. The Keto diet will lower blood sugar levels, and the body will not produce any glucose. You will have more control of the glucose in your blood since the model helps you maintain a more consistent level of blood glucose.

Mental Focus

This is one of the main benefits when you implement the Keto diet. You will find that your energy is replenished, and your brain cells will be more active than before. You will have a sharper brain and be able to focus your attention longer.

Epilepsy Treatment

The Keto diet has been used to treat epilepsy since the 1900s. Both children and adults can get benefits from the Keto diet. As mentioned earlier, the Keto diet plays an important role in the brains' nerve protection since people sticking to the diet use ketones as fuel. Besides, the diet involves intermittent fasting, which is also beneficial for epilepsy patients.

Lower Cholesterol And Blood Pressure

The Keto diet has been shown to improve conditions of cholesterol and triglycerides in the body. Less toxic buildup in the arteries allows blood to flow throughout the body. Low-carb high-fat diets cause a drastic increase in the high-density lipoproteins; thus, improving blood pressure.

Reduce Insulin Resistance

Insulin resistance is the main reason that leads to type II diabetes. The Keto diet will help lower the levels of glucose in the body. This is beneficial because there will be no sugar rush or sudden change in cellular composition.

Chapter 2 Macros, Calories and Nutrition

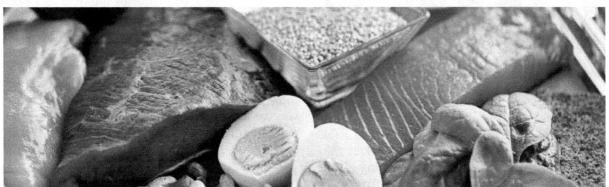

Compared with other diets, you will have a wide array of options to choose from on the Keto diet. The essence of the Keto diet is to get your body into ketosis, and what you need to do is reduce your carbohydrate intake. Except for high-carb foods, you should avoid any proceeded foods that have plenty of artificial additives, let alone junk foods with harmful trans-fats and empty calories.

Some studies have revealed that restricting your calorie intake is beneficial for slowing down the aging process and extending your life span; having balanced macronutrients helps you ease diabetes, polycystic ovary syndrome, and some cancers.

Macros

You might have heard of macros before. Some common phrases include "tracking your macros" or "food that fits your macros." You might ask, What are macros? Could monitoring and counting your macros help you achieve your health goals?

Macros is a term that is short for macronutrients, the main nutrients the body needs, including proteins, fats, and carbohydrates. It is used to show the nutritional information of foods. You can use counting apps or online calculators to calculate macros. Macronutrients are critical in total daily calorie counting. One gram of carbohydrate provides four calories, one gram of protein provides four calories, and one gram of fat provides nine calories. Alcohol is also considered a macronutrient, and it has seven calories per gram, although it has no nutritional value to the body. In this book, we only count proteins, fats, and carbohydrates as macros.

When you follow a diet, you should go beyond counting calories and focus more attention on macros. Depending on your health objectives, you can adjust the ratios of the macros to help you build muscle, lose weight, or maintain weight. If you follow the Keto diet, you will pay attention to net carbohydrates (subtracting the fiber from the total number of carbs) because this will determine how many useful carbohydrates you will intake.

There is another concept, micronutrients, which are the key vitamins and minerals the body needs. Micronutrients are only required in small quantities, but they are essential in all aspects of body functioning from regulating hormones to boosting brain performance.

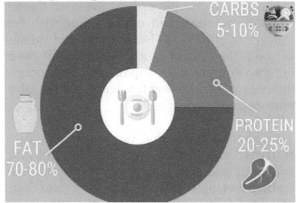

Calories

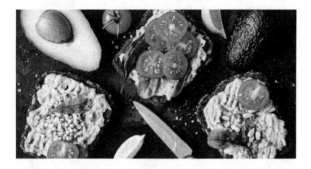

Our resting metabolic rate declines as we age. If we doesn't change what we eat and how much we eat and we keep our same eating habit, it will undoubtedly lead to unwanted weight gain, which will increase the chances of getting certain chronic diseases. The decrease in our metabolic rate is related to the loss of lean body mass. You can completely avoid this by following the Keto diet and maintaining physical activity in order to strengthen your muscles and raise your metabolic rate.

Counting calories differs from tracking macronutrients. The calories-in calories-out approach cannot ensure a balanced ratio of proteins, carbohydrates, and fats for your body. That is why the Keto diet emphasizes the ratio of macros. You will feel completely different when 70% of your calories are coming from carbs instead of fats. However, calorie restriction is necessary for weight loss, and recent research has found that calorie restriction slows down the aging process, prolonging the peoples' lives.

In order to investigate the effects of reducing food intake, Leanne Redman, an endocrinologist at the Pennington Biomedical Research Center at Louisiana State University, along with her colleagues, enrolled 53 healthy men and women between the ages of 21 and 50 and split them into two groups—one group reduced their caloric intake by 15 percent over two years, and the other remained on a regular diet.

The team found that the people who ate a restricted diet lost an average of around nine kilograms and experienced a 10% drop in their resting metabolic rates. When the researchers examined the participants' blood, they also found a reduction in markers of oxidative stress in those who cut down on calories. "After two years, the lower rate of metabolism and level of calorie restriction was linked to a reduction in oxidative damage to cells and tissues," Redman tells.

In general, most women trying to lose weight should aim for 1,500 calories a day, and 1,800 calories in order to maintain their weight. Most men should aim for 1,800 calories to lose weight and 2,100 calories in order to maintain their weight. Everyone is different. You can calculate your basic metabolic value with various online tools, such as MyFitnessPal. For a more accurate way to calculate caloric needs, try an online calorie calculator. You'll find them at USDA Caloric Needs Calculator (fnic.nal.usda.gov) and CalorieKing.com.

The broad effect of calorie restriction on health span and longevity occurs through multiple mechanisms that involve most of the metabolic pathways in tissues and organs. The major effectors are sirtuin deacetylase, AMP - dependent kinase, and PGC-1α. Calorie restriction improves aerobic metabolism by increasing efficient mitochondrial metabolism; thus, lowering the production of endogenous reactive oxygen species while increasing the amount and activity of endogenous antioxidant enzymes. These molecular and physiological effects have also been found with some nutraceuticals and compounds that act as CR mimetics, such as resveratrol, rapamycin, and metformin. CR also affects the lipid composition of membranes by lowering oxidative damage. Further, the study of the mechanisms involved in the prevention of chronic inflammation induced by CR, probably through similar mechanisms to those found in mitochondrial regulation, is increasing and offering new opportunities to understand how CR prevents endogenous damage in an organism.

Unlike other restrictive diets, you can monitor your calories and still enjoy the foods you love. The Keto diet will reduce fat storage in the peripheral and visceral organs, which often causes obesity and other diseases. When your macronutrients are balanced and your calories are restricted, you will feel energized and rejuvenated. However, consult your physician before cutting down your calories.

Nutrition

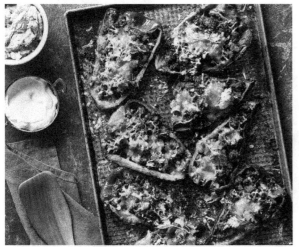

Nutrition is vital for maintaining a healthy biological system. You can live a happy and fulfilling life when you have sufficient nutrition. However, it is imperative to understand that nutrition changes with age, and if you are suffering from nutritional deficiency, then it will bring harmful outcomes. As we all know, nutrition consists of macronutrients and micronutrients. Although people of different age groups need similar macronutrients and micronutrients, this same nutrition has slightly different levels of importance and function in their bodies.

During childhood, the body will require essential nutrients to enable it to grow and develop quickly, both physically and mentally. The food should provide high energy and abundant nutrition in order to enhance a child's cognitive abilities. It is also important to note that children are learning new foods and developing their taste, which will shape their eating habits; therefore, children should be encouraged to consume a wide array of foods. Proteins, for instance, play an essential role in many bodily functions in this age period, including the recovery and repair of tissues. Vitamin A, one of the most essential micronutrients, is vital for boosting the immune system while zinc and iron are necessary for boosting brain ability.

In adolescence, teenagers between 13 and 19 years of age undergo significant changes during puberty. Their bodies become mature gradually, but their bone and muscle growth is very rapid during this stage. For this reason, they will require a diet rich in calcium, such as milk products. Iron is also important for them, and they need to have more meat, chicken, kidney beans, and spinach.

People between 20 and 50 years old usually don't have enough energy and time to care about what they eat because their fast life and work rhythm presents a myriad of challenges. However, this is a time when you are required to maintain a healthy balance in the foods you consume. The body cells are degenerating more than they are being replaced; hence, the need to switch to a healthier diet as well as consider your medical conditions. You should get enough nutrition through proteins, carbohydrates, vitamins, and micronutrients. You must focus on a diet that will help you feel great without disturbing your body in terms of weight and emotional aspects. You need to balance your diet effectively so that you will have the energy to carry out your activities.

When you are over age 50, your body will need more vitamins, minerals, and proteins to help build its cellular structure as well as maintain a balanced diet. Protein in the stage is a vital component in cellular self-rehabilitation and growth. Even though too much protein will lead to gluconeogenesis, we should not neglect the role of protein in ensuring comprehensive nutrition for the body. The body's ability to absorb certain nutrients diminishes; therefore, it is imperative for you to choose a diet that will replenish its nutrients. Eating healthy foods can bring numerous benefits, and it is helpful in slowing down or preventing the aging process. Compared to medical treatment, sticking with the correct diet has unparalleled advantages. It is less expensive and has no side-effects. It can be persisted for a lifetime and can bring vigor and freshness to your life. If you are on a diet that lacks vitamins and minerals, then you should consider adding supplements to your diet. The Keto diet contains comprehensive nutrition that the bodies of seniors need. It is fitting for seniors greatly, as mentioned earlier. There is no need to worry about nutrition when sticking with this diet. Of course, no matter which diet you decide to implement, you should always pay close attention to your body's condition and have physical examinations regularly.

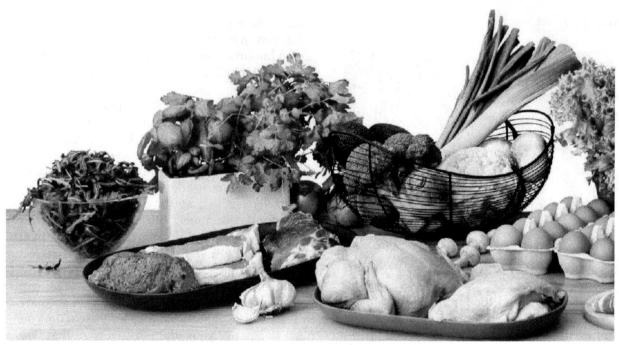

Useful Hints:

Antioxidants

Antioxidants are also called "free-radical scavengers." Antioxidants can prevent or slow damage to cells caused by free radicals. They exist in many vegetables and fruits. Even though there are high-proportion fats, the Keto diet advocates to take in fiber-rich vegetables and low-sugar fruits as all of these provide adequate antioxidants for the human body.

Calcium And Vitamin D

Calcium and vitamin D are two of the most important nutrients for bone health. Seniors are more vulnerable to calcium and vitamin D deficiency as compared to younger people; thus, the intake of these two nutrients are higher in seniors. Both of them can be acquired from nature as well as supplements. For people who are over 50, the IOM-recommended daily allowance is 1000 mg per day of calcium for seniors of age 50. For seniors of age 60, the IOM recommends a daily supplement of 800 to 1000 IU.

Dental Health

It is estimated that over 81% of the adult population has periodontal disease. No matter what diet you are sticking with, oral health affects the taste of a delicious meal. No one is willing to suffer from the pain overnight or not be able to focus under the distraction of pain. Here are some useful tips for oral health care:

◆ Brush your teeth and gums twice a day with a soft-bristled tooth brush and remove the plaque from between your teeth
◆ Floss daily, removing the plaque from the tooth surface. If you don't like to floss, you can choose an alternative, such as inter-dental brushes or electric powered flossers
◆ If you suffer from a dry mouth, try sucking on ice cubes or speaking to your dentist about artificial saliva products
◆ Visit your dentist and hygienist regularly
◆ Eating crunchy vegetables and fruits with their skin on acts as a great natural plaque remover
◆ Quit Smoking
◆ Drink lots of water.

Taste Sensitivity:

Both taste and smell degenerate with the aging process; however, you can revamp them by staying hydrated and reducing the use of salt. Herbs and spices are natural seasonings, and adding them to meals can enhance flavor and help avoid taking in unnecessary salt.

Chapter 3 Getting Started on Keto After 50

People over 50 can feel that there are many changes happening with their bodies. These changes sometimes determine their quality of life. Making dietary changes is an important decision since it will have long-term influence on your body and life. When you are over 50, you might not exercise as much as young people, but the Keto diet caters to this need. On the diet, you don't have to exercise a lot in order to shed unwanted weight. The emphasis is eating whole foods, keeping the right proportion of macros, and controlling your calories according to your basic metabolic value. We should get some background information about the Keto diet before we go into the many details about it.

Seniors over 50 may take time to adjust to dietary changes, but everyone is different. Someone may take a shorter amount of time than others. You might experience headaches, nausea, fatigue, or dizziness; however, this is not the reason to quit. Don't be worried or disappointed when you face various challenges in adapting to the diet; this is very common. We should find resolutions actively in order to achieve our target.

The guidelines for starting the Keto diet are as follows:

Decrease Carbohydrates intake

This might seem simple, but it is the most intractable aspect of the Keto diet. The essence of the Keto diet is to reduce the intake of carbohydrates while boosting fats and proteins. In the beginning, you can decrease your carb intake gradually in order to allow your body to adapt to the changes.

Prepare Fatty Meals

When it comes to fatty meals, it does not mean all kinds of fats. The fats you choose should include those with adequate unsaturated fats. Besides, preparing yummy snacks with rich fats is one of the most effective tricks to having success on the Keto diet. It's satisfying to have all kinds of meats and fats in a diet; however, what you should be watchful of is not exceeding the calorie value you set for yourself.

Do Not Eat Too Much Proteins

Your daily protein intake should not exceed 25% of all of your daily calorie intake. Eating too much protein will cause gluconeogenesis, which is the production of glucose and it will slow down the process of getting into ketosis.

Do Not Restrict Calories Before The Body Adopts To The Diet

It is important that as much as you are looking for a high-protein diet, you should always allow your body to adapt as you cut calories slowly until you are ready to handle it.

Monitor Calories

One of the best ways to adapt to a new diet is by tracking your macros and calorie intake. This will help your body replenish itself and generate more cells as your body obtains sufficient daily nutritional intake. You should adjust until your body is ready to adapt to the state of ketosis.

Get into Ketosis

Many people over 50 will encounter obstacles as they get into ketosis. If you face the same difficulty, you can:

Limit your carb intake to 20 to 50 net grams per day; thus, lowering your blood sugar and insulin levels, leading to the release of stored fatty acids that your liver converts into ketones.

Consume coconut oil, which provides your body with MCTs that are quickly absorbed and converted into ketone bodies by your liver. Engaging in physical activity can increase ketone levels during carb restriction.

This effect may be enhanced by working out in a fasted state. Consuming at least 60% of calories from fat will help boost your ketone levels.

Choose a variety of healthy fats from both plant and animal sources. Fasting, intermittent fasting, and a "fat fast" can all help you get into ketosis relatively quickly.

Consuming too little of protein can lead to muscle mass loss, whereas excessive protein intake may suppress ketone production.

Best Ketogenic Food List For Seniors

The secret to the successful implementation of the Keto diet is to have a good plan. When you have a good plan, you can easily stick with it and overcome any challenge that may arise during the process. There are essential foods that you can consume in order to get your body into ketosis as well as foods that you should avoid in order to prevent getting out of ketosis.

Fats:

Oil:
- Almond oil
- Avocado oil
- Butter (grass-fed dairy)
- Cacao butter/oil
- Canola oil
- Chicken fat (schmaltz) - free-range
- Coconut oil
- Duck fat (free-range)
- Flaxseed oil
- Ghee (grass-fed)
- Goose fat (free-range)
- Hazelnut oil
- Hemp seed oil
- Lard (pasture-raised)
- Macadamia nut oil
- MCT oil
- Olive oil
- Palm fruit oil
- Palm kernel oil
- Tallow/suet (grass-fed)
- Walnut oil

Beef:
- Brisket
- Ground beef (30% fat)
- Liver pate
- New York strip steak
- Pepperoni
- Porterhouse steak
- Prime rib steak
- Rib roast
- Rib-eye
- Ribs
- Roast
- Sausage
- Skirt steak
- T-bone steak

Power Foods:
- Avocados
- Beef tallow
- Coconut oil
- Dark chocolate (100% raw cacao and/or sugar-free)
- Flax seeds

Nuts/Seeds:
- Almonds
- Brazil nuts
- Cashews
- Chia seeds
- Coconut
- Hazelnuts
- Hemp seeds
- Macadamia nuts
- Pecans
- Pine nuts
- Pistachios
- Pumpkin seeds
- Sesame seeds
- Sunflower seeds
- Walnuts

Nut or Seed Foods:
- Almond butter
- Brazil nut butter
- Coconut butter
- Hazelnut butter
- Hemp seed butter
- Macadamia nut butter
- Pecan butter
- Sunflower seed butter
- Tahini
- Walnut butter

Other Whole Foods:
- Avocados
- Bacon
- Olives

Protein:

Power foods:
- Eggs
- Liver
- Pacific salmon (wild-caught)
- Sardines

Pork:
- Bacon (side or slab)
- Ground pork
- Pepperoni
- Pork dust (ground pork rinds)
- Pork rinds
- Pork shoulder
- Sausage
- Spare ribs

Seafood:
- Crab
- Herring
- Lobster
- Mackerel
- Marine collagen
- Salmon (wild-caught)
- Sardines
- Squid
- Trout

Lamb:
- Loin
- Sirloin
- Rib chops

Wild side:
- Bison
- Elk
- Goat
- Mutton

Poultry:
- Eggs
- Liver pate
- Skin
- Thighs (with skin)
- Whole (with skin)
- Wings (with skin)

Plant-Based Proteins:
- Amaranth
- Hemp seeds
- Legumes
- Millet
- Oatmeal
- Peas
- Plant protein powder
- Quinoa
- Spirulina
- Tempeh
- Tofu
- Wild rice

Carbohydrates:
Power Foods:
- Vegetables (see here)
- Broccoli
- Garlic
- Kale
- Fruits
- Avocados
- Blueberries
- Raw coconut

Light Carbs Enjoy Liberally
Vegetables:
- Artichoke hearts
- Arugula
- Asparagus
- Bell peppers (green)
- Bok choy
- Broccoli
- Cabbage
- Capers
- Cauliflower
- Celery
- Chard
- Collards
- Cucumbers
- Daikon
- Eggplant
- Endive/escarole
- Fennel
- Garlic
- Kohlrabi
- Lettuce
- Mushrooms
- Okra
- Radishes
- Rhubarb
- Shallots
- Spinach
- Swiss chard
- Turnips
- Zucchini
- Fruits
- Olives
- Tomatoes

For higher carbs, eat sparingly.
Vegetables:
- Artichoke
- Beets
- Brussels sprouts
- Buttercup squash
- Carrots
- Celeriac
- Jicama
- Kale
- Onion
- Pumpkin
- Rutabaga
- Spaghetti squash

Fruits:
- Blackberries
- Cranberries
- Lemons
- Limes
- Raspberries
- Strawberries
- Watermelon

Drinks:
- Almond milk
- Coconut milk, light or full-fat
- Coffee
- Soda sweetened with stevia
- Sparkling water
- Tea

Sweeteners:
- Erythritol
- Monk fruit extractor han guo
- Stevia, alcohol-free
- Xylitol

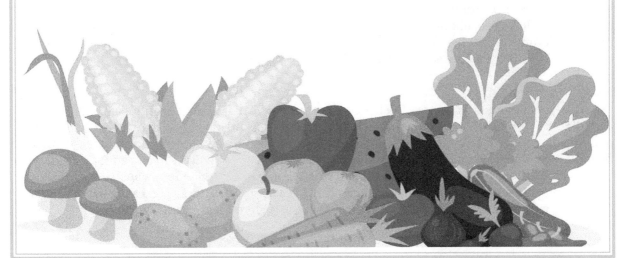

Foods to Avoid When On Keto Diet over 50

There are foods that you should avoid if you are on a keto diet after 50 years.

Keto Foods To Avoid

Low Fat / High Carb (Based On Net Carbs)

Meats & Meat Alternatives
- Deli meat (some, not all)
- Hot dogs (with fillers)
- Sausage (with fillers)
- Seitan
- Tofu

Dairy
- Almond milk (sweetened)
- Coconut milk (sweetened)
- Milk
- Soy milk (regular)
- Yogurt (regular)

Nuts & Seeds
- Cashews
- Chestnuts
- Pistachios

Fruits & Vegetables
- Apples
- Apricots
- Artichokes
- Bananas
- Beans (all varieties)
- Boysenberries
- Burdock root
- Butternut squash
- Cantaloupe
- Cherries
- Chickpeas
- Corn
- Currants
- Dates
- Edamame
- Eggplant
- Elderberries
- Gooseberries
- Grapes
- Honeydew melon
- Huckleberries
- Kiwifruits
- Leeks
- Mangos
- Oranges
- Parsnips
- Peaches
- Peas
- Pineapples
- Plantains
- Plums
- Potatoes
- Prunes
- Raisins
- Sweet potatoes
- Taro root
- Turnips
- Water chestnuts
- Winter squash
- Yams

Troubleshooting

Generally, the Keto diet is safe for most people; however, I suggest to consult your doctor and make a comprehensive physical examination before executing the Keto diet. There are some symptoms you may experience with the Keto diet, such as dehydration, fatigue, insomnia, frequent urination, diarrhea, and low metabolic activity. Some people experience fewer symptoms while others experience more. With some people, symptoms might only last for a short time while for other people, they might last longer. In either case, these symptoms will disappear in about two weeks.

Keto Flu

This is a natural reaction that the body will undergo when switching from a high-carb to a low-carb diet. The symptoms of this flu include brain fog, insomnia, irritability, sugar cravings, poor focus, and muscle soreness. Keto flu affects some people more than others; however, you can overcome it by drinking enough water and cycling some carbs one day out of the week. You can take in salt and bouillon cubes in order to supply sodium, along with red meats, spinach, mushrooms, and avocados in order to supply potassium. You can also take in hemp seeds, seaweed, and magnesium supplements in order to supply magnesium. Finally, don't forget to get enough rest and exercise regularly.

Keto Rash

Keto rash is a rare form of dermatitis or skin inflammation. It is an itchy and uncomfortable rash that develops on the upper body. Keto rash appears as raised, red, itchy papules on the skin. Skin redness or erythema can be more difficult to detect on dark skin. The minority of people on the Keto diet will experience keto rash. However, this can be averted by eating some carbs, avoiding irritants, such as wool or strong detergents, avoiding touching the rash whenever possible, moisturizing the area several times a day, washing the skin gently, and avoiding excessive rubbing.

Insomnia

There is no research on the effects of the Keto diet and sleep problems; however, according to recent data, many people report waking up in the middle of the night when they are on the Keto diet. If you find that you are having trouble sleeping at night and you are on the Keto diet, then you should do the following: take a teaspoon of raw honey, which will provide you with adequate carbs in order to allow you to sleep adequately.

Bad breath: Acetone is a ketone produced at a high level in ketosis, and it is responsible for bad breath. In order to curb this problem, brush your teeth and tongue often, and chew sugar-free gum.

Appetite suppression: Hunger decreases in ketosis because fats burn slower than carbohydrates. You may feel fuller for a longer period of time with reduced appetite.

Short-term fatigue: The depletion of electrolytes at the start may lead to weakness and tiredness; however, staying focused on the diet and boosting your electrolytes eventually curbs this problem.

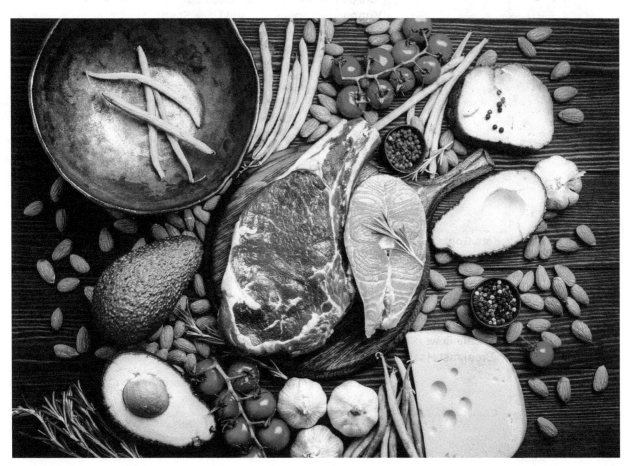

28 Day Meal Plan

	Breakfast	Lunch	Dinner	Desserts
1	Easy Smoked Salmon Roll-Ups	Tomato And Eggplant With Rich Chicken Thighs	Lamb Chops With Dry Red Wine	Banana Creamy Fat Bombs
		Kale Salad With The Bacon And Blue Cheese	Yogurt, Cheese, And Dill Stuffed Tomato	
2	Baked Cream Cheese Muffins	Hot Pork And Bell Pepper In Lettuce	Garlicky Parmesan Salmon With Asparagus	Frozen Blueberry Keto Fat Bombs
		Cauliflower An Pecan Casserole With Pecans	Spicy And Sour Chicken Stew	
3	Bacon And Egg Avocado Breakfast Wrap	Crispy Crackers With Sesame Seeds	Beef Salad With Vegetables	Vanilla And Cream Custard
		Crispy Prosciutto-Wrapped Haddock Fillets	Smoked Salmon And Leek Soup	
4	Blueberry Nutty Oatmeal	Jambalaya Broth	Salmon And Lettuce Salad	Strawberry Cheesecake
		Jerk Pork	Chicken And Avocado Wrapped Lettuce	
5	Mushroom And Spinach Cheese Frittata	Beef And Pumpkin Stew	Cauliflower Mash	Lemony Cheesecake
		Cauliflower And Cashew Nut Salad	Braised Chicken, Bacon, And Mushrooms	
6	Keto Goat Cheese Salmon Fat Bombs	Garlicky Lamb Leg With Rosemary	Niçoise Salad	Cocoa Fudge
		Garlicky Parmesan Salmon With Asparagus	Lamb And Tomato Curry	
7	Cauliflower Breakfast Hash	Easy Cheesy Spinach Balls	Lamb Curry Stew	Peanut Butter Blackberry Bars
		Baked Salmon With Mayo Sauce	Aromatic Roasted Duck	

8	Crab Salad Stuffed Avocados	Herbed Eggs With Butter	Beef, Eggplant, Zucchini, And Baby Spinach Lasagna	Easy Berry Bites
		Greek Salad With Vinaigrette Salad Dressing	Prawns Salad With Mixed Lettuce Greens	
9	Low-Carb Coconut Bread	Crispy Brussels Sprouts With Bacon Slices	Buttered Scallops With Herbs	Matcha Balls With Coconut
		Italian Sausage, Zucchini, Eggplant, And Tomato Ratatouille	Creamy Cauliflower And Celery Soup With Crisp Bacon	
10	Bacon And Egg Avocado Breakfast Wrap	Lemony Anchovy Butter With Steaks	Turkey Meatloaf	Easy Sesame Cookies
		Cauliflower, Shrimp And Cucumber Salad	Spicy Sausage And Chicken Scarpariello	
11	Blueberry Nutty Oatmeal	Tender Zucchini With Cheese	Cheesy Kale Stuffed Zucchini	Matcha And Macadamia Brownies
		Ricotta, Prosciutto, And Spinach Chicken Rollatini	Garlicky Lamb Leg With Rosemary	
12	Mushroom And Spinach Cheese Frittata	Cheesy Crackers With Guacamole	Turkey Meatloaf	Lemony Cheesecake
		Slow Cooker Creamed Vegetables	Smoothy Green Soup	
13	Keto Goat Cheese Salmon Fat Bombs	Rich Cucumber And Avocado Soup With Tomato	Pork Rind Green Beans With Parmesan Cheese	Strawberry Cheesecake
		Ricotta, Prosciutto, And Spinach Chicken Rollatini	Mushroom, Spinach, And Onion Stuffed Meatloaf	
14	Cauliflower Breakfast Hash	Roasted And Buttery Radishes	Cherry Tomato Gratin	Cocoa Fudge
		Fish Curry With Kale And Cilantro	Cold Avocado And Crab Soup	
15	Crab Salad Stuffed Avocados	Sauerkraut And Sausage Soup	Chicken Caprese	Banana Creamy Fat Bombs
		Bacon, Beef, And Pecan Patties	Simple Sautéed Asparagus Spears With Walnuts	

16	Low-Carb Coconut Bread	Sweet And Buttery Red Cabbage	Baked Pork Rind Zucchini Halves	Easy Berry Bites
		Chicken Thigh And Tomato Braise	Spicy Chicken Breasts	
17	Easy Smoked Salmon Roll-Ups	Turkey, Baby Spinach, And Zucchini Frittata	Italian Flavor Herbed Pork Chops	Matcha And Macadamia Brownies
		Simple Sautéed Asparagus Spears With Walnuts	Creamy Chicken Pot Pie Soup	
18	Baked Cream Cheese Muffins	Chicken Salad And Cucumber Bites	Tomato And Artichoke Caponata With Grilled Salmon Fillets	Cocoa Fudge
		Zucchini Carbonara	Seared Squid Salad With Red Chili Dressing	
19	Keto Goat Cheese Salmon Fat Bombs	Poached Egg Salad With Lettuce And Olives	Grilled Sea Bass With Olive Sauce	Easy Sesame Cookies
		Braised Beef Shanks And Dry Red Wine	Spinach And Olive Stuffed Chicken With Mozzarella	
20	Cauliflower Breakfast Hash	Jalapeno Turkey Bites With Tomato Slices	Shrimp, Tomato, And Avocado Salad	Frozen Blueberry Keto Fat Bombs
		Cheesy And Buttered Salmon	Veggie Chili With Avocado Cream	
21	Low-Carb Coconut Bread	Browned Frittata With Ham	Bacon Avocado Salad	Peanut Butter Blackberry Bars
		Browned Salmon With Tomato Salad	Lamb And Tomato Curry	
22	Bacon And Egg Avocado Breakfast Wrap	Fried Halibut With Citrus Sauce	Smoked Salmon And Leek Soup	Vanilla And Cream Custard
		Greek Salad With Vinaigrette Salad Dressing	Lemony Anchovy Butter With Steaks	
23	Mushroom And Spinach Cheese Frittata	Fried Pork Rind Crusted Salmon Cakes	Smoothy Green Soup	Banana Creamy Fat Bombs
		Herbed Eggs With Butter	Chicken Thigh And Tomato Braise	

24	Keto Goat Cheese Salmon Fat Bombs	Lemony And Spicy Shrimp	Crispy Crackers With Sesame Seeds	Peanut Butter Blackberry Bars
		Poached Egg Salad With Lettuce And Olives	Braised Chicken, Bacon, And Mushrooms	
25	Baked Cream Cheese Muffins	Cauliflower, Shrimp And Cucumber Salad	Cauliflower An Pecan Casserole With Pecans	Matcha And Macadamia Brownies
		Cheesy And Buttered Salmon	Spicy Sausage And Chicken Scarpariello	
26	Easy Smoked Salmon Roll-Ups	Cold Avocado And Crab Soup	Fried Halibut With Citrus Sauce	Frozen Blueberry Keto Fat Bombs
		Braised Beef Shanks And Dry Red Wine	Salmon And Lettuce Salad	
27	Cauliflower Breakfast Hash	Aromatic Roasted Duck	Pork Rind Green Beans With Parmesan Cheese	Cocoa Fudge
		Sauerkraut And Sausage Soup	Lamb And Tomato Curry	
28	Low-Carb Coconut Bread	Smoked Salmon And Leek Soup	Fried Pork Rind Crusted Salmon Cakes	Banana Creamy Fat Bombs
		Beef, Eggplant, Zucchini, And Baby Spinach Lasagna	Jambalaya Broth	

APPETIZERS AND SNACKS

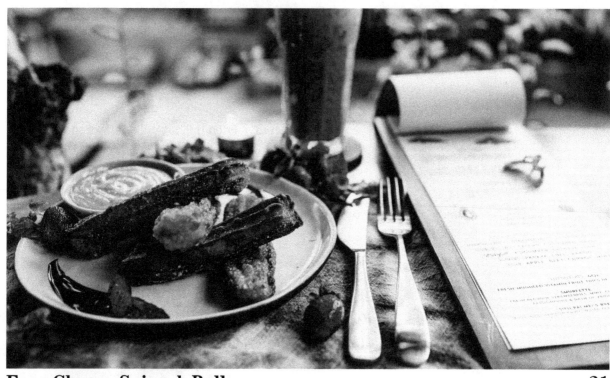

EASY CHEESY SPINACH BALLS

Macros: Fat 79% | Protein 15% | Carbs 6%

Prep time: 10 minutes | Cook time: 12 minutes | Serves 8

1. Preheat the oven to 350°F (180°C). Line a baking sheet with parchment paper and set aside.
2. Purée all ingredients in a food processor until creamy and whipped.
3. Transfer the mixture to a large bowl. Cover, and refrigerate to chill for about 10 minutes.
4. Take the bowl out of the refrigerator, then start the balls by using a cookie scoop to scoop out equal-sized amounts of the mixture and form into balls with your palm. Arrange the balls on the parchment-lined baking sheet.
5. Bake in the preheated oven for about 10 to 12 minutes until cooked through.
6. Allow to cool for 8 minutes before serving.

TIP: You can cover and freeze the unbaked spinach balls in the freezer for up to 1 month.

PER SERVING
calories: 60 | fat: 5.3g | protein: 2.2g | net carbs: 0.9g

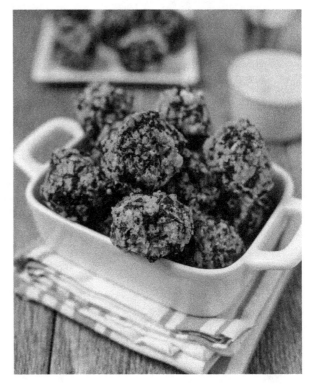

Ingredients:

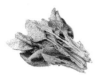

8 ounces (227 g) spinach

⅓ cup ricotta cheese, crumbled

3 tablespoons heavy cream

2 tablespoons butter, melted

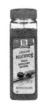

¼ teaspoon nutmeg

¼ teaspoon pepper

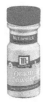

1 tablespoon onion powder

1 teaspoon garlic powder

⅓ cup Parmesan cheese

2 eggs, whisked

1 cup almond flour

HERBED EGGS WITH BUTTER

Macros: Fat 79% | Protein 18% | Carbs 3%

Prep time: 10 minutes | Cook time: 10 minutes | Serves 4

1. In a large skillet over medium heat, melt the butter and coconut oil.
2. Toss in the garlic and thyme, and cook for about 30 seconds until fragrant. Add the cilantro and parsley, stirring, and cook for 2 to 3 minutes until just wilted.
3. Gently crack the eggs one at a time into the skillet. Reduce the heat and cook for an additional 4 to 6 minutes until the eggs are just set. Sprinkle with the cumin, cayenne pepper, salt, and black pepper.
4. Remove from the heat to four serving plates, then serve.

TIP: You can store the leftovers in an airtight container in the fridge for 2 to 3 days.

PER SERVING
calories: 293.3 | fat: 25.7g | protein: 13g | net carbs: 2.51g

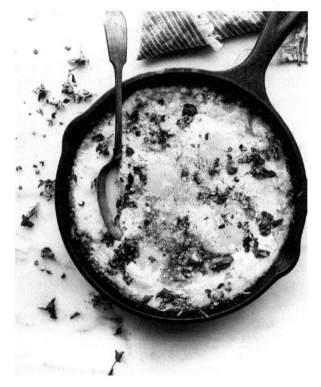

Ingredients:

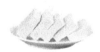

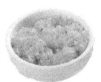

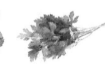

| 2 tablespoons butter | 1 tablespoon coconut oil | 2 garlic cloves, minced | 1 teaspoon fresh thyme | ½ cup cilantro, chopped | ½ cup parsley, chopped |

| 4 eggs | ¼ teaspoon cumin | ¼ teaspoon cayenne pepper | Salt and black pepper, to taste | |

ROASTED AND BUTTERY RADISHES

Macros: Fat 93% | Protein 2% | Carbs 5%

Prep time: 10 minutes | Cook time: 15 minutes | Serves 2

1. Preheat the oven to 450°F (235°C). Line a baking sheet with parchment paper and set aside.
2. Add the olive oil and radishes in a medium bowl. Toss well until the radishes are coated thoroughly. Sprinkle with salt and pepper.
3. Spread the radishes around the prepared baking sheet without overlapping.
4. Roast in the preheated oven for about 15 minutes, stirring halfway through the cooking time, or until tender.
5. Meanwhile, melt the butter in a saucepan over medium heat. Add a pinch of salt, stirring constantly and swirling the melted butter until brown flecks appear, for about 3 minutes.
6. Remove the radishes from the oven to two plates. Drizzle them with the brown butter, then serve topped with the fresh parsley.

TIP: Don't overcook the butter in the saucepan, or it will turn dark.

PER SERVING
calories: 186.5 | fat: 19.3g | protein: 1.2g | net carbs: 2g | fiber: 2g

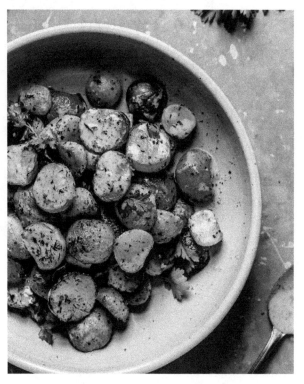

Ingredients:

 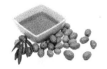   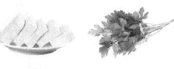

| 2 cups radishes, halved | 1 tablespoon olive oil | Pink Himalayan salt, to taste | Freshly ground black pepper, to taste | 2 tablespoons butter | 1 tablespoon fresh parsley, chopped |

PORK RIND GREEN BEANS WITH PARMESAN CHEESE

Macros: Fat 76% | Protein 14% | Carbs 10%

Prep time: 5 minutes | Cook time: 15 minutes | Serves 2

1. Preheat the oven to 450°F (235°C). Line a baking sheet with parchment paper and set aside.
2. Mix together the green beans, pork rinds, Parmesan cheese, olive oil, salt, and pepper in a medium bowl. Toss to coat well.
3. Arrange the coated green beans mixture on the baking sheet, close together.
4. Roast in the preheated oven for about 15 minutes until the cheese has a beautiful golden color, giving a good stir or shaking the pan halfway through.
5. Remove from the oven and serve on plates.

TIP: To add additional zest to the dish, you can try any flavor of pork rinds.

PER SERVING
calories: 182.9 | fat: 15.3g | protein: 6.2g | net carbs: 4.8g | fiber: 3g

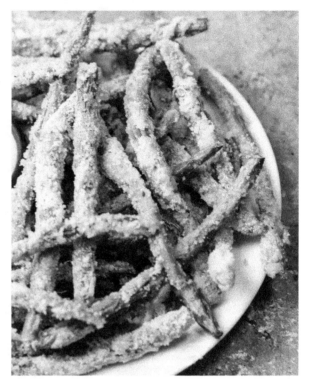

Ingredients:

   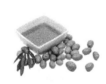

| ½ pound (227 g) fresh green beans | 2 tablespoons crushed pork rinds | 1 tablespoon Parmesan cheese, shredded | 2 tablespoons olive oil | Pink Himalayan salt, to taste | Freshly ground black pepper, to taste |

CHEESY CRACKERS WITH GUACAMOLE

Macros: Fat 76% | Protein 19% | Carbs 5%

Prep time: 5 minutes | Cook time: 5 minutes | Serves 4

1. Preheat the oven to 350°F (180°C) and line a baking sheet with parchment paper.
2. In a bowl, stir together the Parmesan cheese, paprika, and Italian seasoning. Scoop tablespoon-sized mounds of the cheese mixture onto the baking sheet, evenly spaced but not too close together, and press each mound down slightly.
3. Bake in the preheated oven for about 5 minutes until the edges are golden brown.
4. Remove the crackers from the heat and set aside on a plate to cool.
5. Make the guacamole: Using a fork, mash the avocado in a large bowl. Add the tomato, tabasco sauce, and cilantro, then continue mashing until the mixture is mostly smooth. Sprinkle with the salt.
6. Serve the crackers with the guacamole on the side.

TIP: The guacamole can be made ahead, but don't add the cilantro before serving.

PER SERVING
calories: 268.7 | fat: 22.7g | protein: 12.9g | net carbs: 3.2g

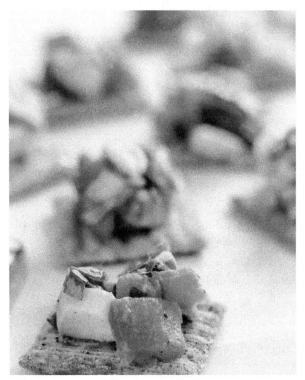

CRACKERS:

| 1 cup grated Parmesan cheese | ¼ teaspoon sweet paprika | ¼ teaspoon Italian seasoning |

GUACAMOLE:

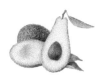

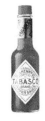

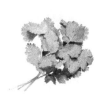

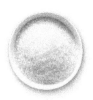

2 soft avocados, pitted and scooped   1 tomato, chopped   1 teaspoon low-carb tabasco sauce   1 teaspoon cilantro, chopped   Salt, to taste

BROWNED FRITTATA WITH HAM

Macros: Fat 78% | Protein 19% | Carbs 3%

Prep time: 10 minutes | Cook time: 10 minutes | Serves 4

1. Preheat the oven to 400°F (205°C). Lightly grease a baking dish with melted butter and set aside.
2. In a medium bowl, beat the eggs, melted butter, almond milk, salt, and pepper until smooth and frothy.
3. Add the ham pieces and stir to combine. Slowly pour the mixture into the prepared baking dish. Scatter the cheese and green onion on top of the mixture.
4. Bake in the preheated oven for about 10 minutes until lightly browned around the edges and the eggs are completely set.
5. Allow to cool for 8 minutes before slicing into wedges.

TIP: To make this a complete meal, serve it with keto vanilla milkshake.

PER SERVING
calories: 304.3 | fat: 26.3g | protein: 14.6g | net carbs: 2.3g

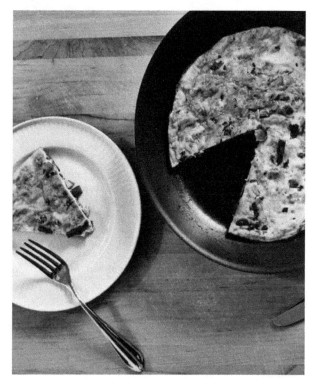

Ingredients:

2 tablespoons melted butter, plus more for greasing the baking dish

8 eggs

8 ounces (227 g) ham, cut into small pieces

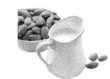

2 tablespoons almond milk

1 green onion, chopped

1 cup shredded Cheddar cheese

Salt and black pepper, to taste

BAKED PORK RIND ZUCCHINI HALVES

Macros: Fat 76% | Protein 15% | Carbs 9%

Prep time: 5 minutes | Cook time: 25 minutes | Serves 2

1. Preheat the oven to 400°F (205°C) and line a baking sheet with aluminum foil. Set aside.
2. Make the toppings: Mix together the pork rinds, melted butter, Parmesan cheese, garlic, salt, and pepper in a large bowl. Toss to combine well.
3. Arrange the halved zucchini, cut-side up, on the baking sheet. Spoon equal portions of the pork rind mixture onto zucchini halves. Drizzle the top of each zucchini half with olive oil.
4. Bake in the preheated oven until golden brown, about 20 minutes. Broil for 3 to 5 minutes until crisp, if needed.
5. Remove from the oven and serve hot.

TIP: You can hollow out the zucchini halves with a spoon for more toppings.

PER SERVING
calories: 243.5 | fat: 20.3g | protein: 9.1g | net carbs: 5.7g | fiber: 2g

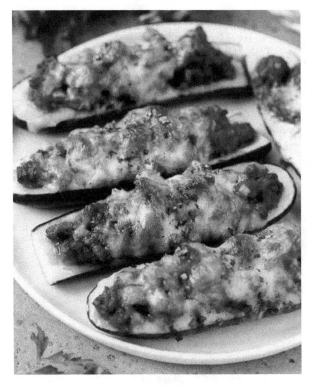

TOPPINGS:

¼ cup pork rinds, crushed

2 tablespoons melted butter

¼ cup Parmesan cheese, shredded

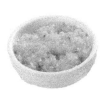
2 garlic cloves, minced

Pink Himalayan salt, to taste

Freshly ground black pepper, to taste

2 medium zucchini, halved lengthwise and seeded

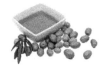
1 teaspoon olive oil, for drizzling

CHICKEN SALAD AND CUCUMBER BITES

Macros: Fat 67% | Protein 28% | Carbs 5%

Prep time: 15 minutes | Cook time: 0 minutes | Serves 2

1. Make the salad: Combine the chicken, pecans, celery, mayo, salt, and pepper in a medium bowl. Toss well and set aside.
2. Divide the cucumber slices between two plates and sprinkle with the salt.
3. To serve, top each plate evenly of cucumber slices with the chicken salad.

TIP: For additional zest and crunch, you can cover, and refrigerate them for 1 day before serving.

PER SERVING
calories: 327.9 | fat: 24.3g | protein: 23.2g | net carbs: 4.1g | fiber: 3g

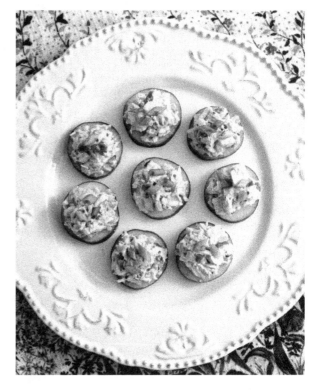

SALAD:

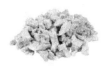

1 cup cooked chicken breast, diced

¼ cup chopped pecans

¼ cup diced celery

2 tablespoons mayonnaise

Pink Himalayan salt, to taste

Freshly ground black pepper, to taste

1 cucumber, peeled and cut into ¼-inch slices

GRILLED SEA BASS WITH OLIVE SAUCE

Macros: Fat 58% | Protein 39% | Carbs 3%

Prep time: 15 minutes | Cook time: 10 minutes | Serves 4

1. Preheat the grill to high heat.
2. Stir together 1 tablespoon olive oil, chili pepper, and salt in a bowl. Brush both sides of each sea bass fillet generously with the mixture.
3. Grill the fillets on the preheated grill for about 5 to 6 minutes on each side until lightly browned.
4. Meanwhile, warm the remaining olive oil in a skillet over medium heat. Add the green olives, lemon juice, and salt. Cook for 3 to 4 minutes until the sauce is heated through.
5. Transfer the fillets to four serving plates, then pour the sauce over them. Serve warm.

TIP: To make this recipe easy, you can buy cooked fish fillets in the market.

PER SERVING
calories: 246.7 | fat: 15.9g | protein: 24.2g | net carbs: 1.7g

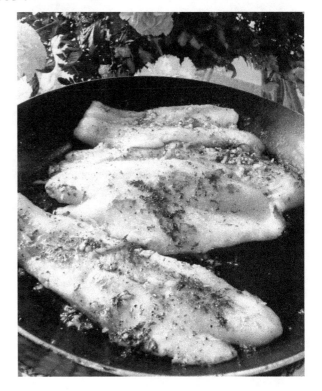

FISH:

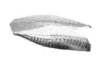

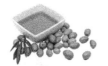

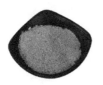

| 4 sea bass fillets | 2 tablespoons olive oil, divided | A pinch of chili pepper | Salt, to taste |

OLIVE SAUCE:

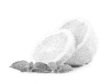

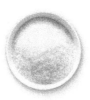

| 1 tablespoon green olives, pitted and sliced | 1 lemon, juiced | Salt, to taste |

CRISPY BRUSSELS SPROUTS WITH BACON SLICES

Macros: Fat 67% | Protein 23% | Carbs 10%

Prep time: 5 minutes | Cook time: 25 minutes | Serves 2

1. Preheat the oven to 400°F (205°C). Line a baking sheet with parchment paper and set aside.
2. Toss the Brussels sprouts in the olive oil in a medium bowl. Add the salt, pepper, and red pepper flakes, and mix well.
3. Spread out the Brussels sprouts and bacon pieces on the prepared baking sheet in a single layer.
4. Roast in the preheated oven for about 25 minutes until the Brussels sprouts have a perfectly crispy outside, giving a good stir or shaking the pan halfway through.
5. Divide the Brussels sprouts and bacon between two serving plates. Serve topped with shredded Parmesan cheese.

TIP: The Parmesan cheese can be ditched if you want to make this meal dairy-free.

PER SERVING
calories: 248.6 | fat: 18.2g | protein: 14.1g | net carbs: 7.1g | fiber: 5g

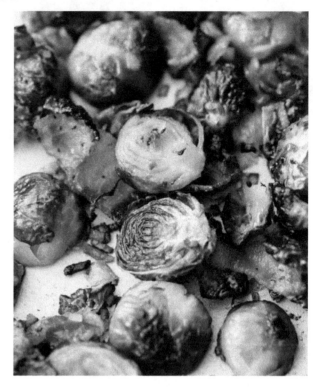

Ingredients:

½ pound (227 g) Brussels sprouts, cleaned, trimmed, and halved

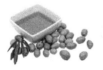

1 tablespoon olive oil

Pink Himalayan salt, to taste

Freshly ground black pepper, to taste

1 teaspoon red pepper flakes

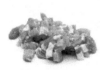

6 bacon slices, cut into 1-inch pieces.

1 tablespoon Parmesan cheese, shredded

JALAPENO TURKEY BITES WITH TOMATO SLICES

Macros: Fat 56% | Protein 34% | Carbs 10%

Prep time: 10 minutes | Cook time: 0 minutes | Serves 4

1. In a bowl, mix together the turkey ham, jalapeño pepper, mayo, mustard, salt, and pepper.
2. Spread out the tomato slices on four serving plates, then top each plate with a spoonful of the turkey ham mixture.
3. Serve garnished with chopped parsley.

TIP: To add more flavors to this meal, you can sprinkle with dill or basil.

PER SERVING
calories: 250 | fat: 15.5g | protein: 21.2g | net carbs: 6.4g

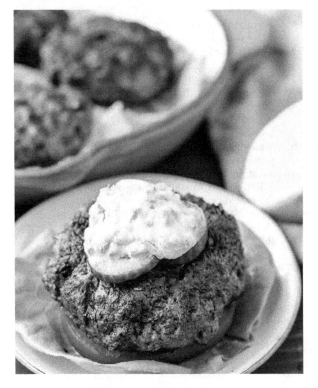

Ingredients:

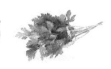

1 cup turkey ham, chopped	¼ jalapeño pepper, minced	¼ cup mayonnaise	⅓ tablespoon Dijon mustard	4 tomatoes, sliced	1 tablespoon parsley, chopped

Salt and black pepper, to taste

CRISPY CRACKERS WITH SESAME SEEDS

Macros: Fat 77% | Protein 17% | Carbs 6%

Prep time: 10 minutes | Cook time: 12 minutes | Serves 4

1. Preheat the oven to 350°F (180°C). Line a baking sheet with parchment paper and set aside.
2. In a bowl, combine the flour, baking powder, Gruyère cheese, and salt. Stir well and set aside.
3. Beat the eggs, yogurt, and melted butter in another bowl until creamy.
4. Slowly pour the egg mixture into the bowl of dry ingredients, whisking constantly, or until it forms a smooth batter.
5. Make the crackers: Using a soup spoon, scoop portions of the batter onto the prepared baking sheet and flatten each to about 1/16-inch thickness with a rolling pin. Scatter the sesame seeds over the crackers.
6. Bake in the preheated oven until golden brown, about 12 minutes.
7. Remove from the oven and serve warm.

TIP: Remember to leave 2-inch intervals between each crackers when placing them onto the baking sheet.

PER SERVING
calories: 384 | fat: 32.8g | protein: 16.6g | net carbs: 5.6g

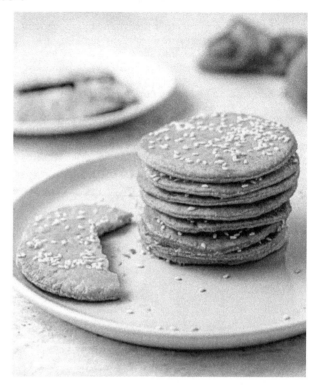

Ingredients:

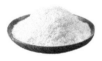
⅓ cup almond flour

1 teaspoon baking powder

1¼ cups Gruyère cheese, grated

Salt, to taste

5 eggs

⅓ cup plain Greek yogurt

⅓ cup butter, melted

1 tablespoon sesame seeds

BREAKFAST

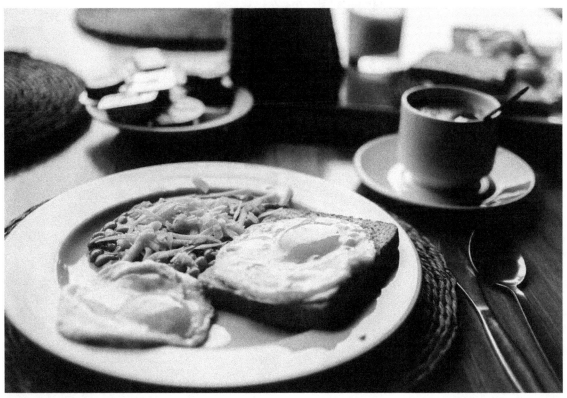

EASY SMOKED SALMON ROLL-UPS

Macros: Fat 74% | Protein 21% | Carbs 5%

Prep time: 25 minutes | Cook time: 0 minutes | Serves 2

1. In a food processor, pulse the cream cheese, mustard, scallions, lemon zest, salt, and pepper until combined thoroughly.
2. Make the roll-ups: Lay the smoked salmon slices on a clean work surface. Divide the cream cheese mixture among the salmon slices and evenly spread it all over, then roll them up. Transfer the roll-ups, seam-side down, to a plate.
3. Serve immediately, or cover with plastic wrap and refrigerate for 1 hour before serving.

TIP: The scallions can be replaced with chopped fresh dill.

PER SERVING
calories: 270 | fat: 22.3g | protein: 14.2g | net carbs: 3.2g | fiber: 1g

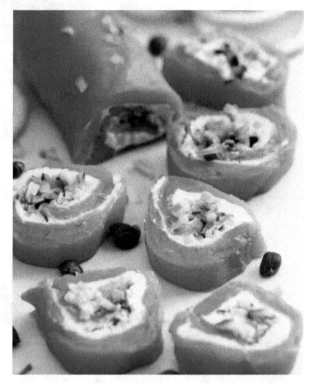

Ingredients:

4 ounces (113 g) cream cheese, at room temperature

1 teaspoon Dijon mustard

2 tablespoons chopped scallions, white and green parts

1 teaspoon grated lemon zest

Pink Himalayan salt, to taste

Freshly ground black pepper, to taste

1 (4-ounce/ 113-g) package cold and smoked salmon (about 12 slices)

BAKED CREAM CHEESE MUFFINS

Macros: Fat 81% | Protein 12% | Carbs 7%

Prep time: 10 minutes | Cook time: 12 minutes | Makes 6 muffins

1. Preheat the oven to 400°F (205°C). Grease 6 muffin tin cups with melted butter and set aside.
2. Combine the baking powder and almond flour in a bowl. Stir well and set aside.
3. Stir together 4 tablespoons melted butter, eggs, shredded cheese, and cream cheese in a separate bowl.
4. Add the dry mixture into the egg mixture, then using a hand mixer to beat until it is creamy and well blended.
5. Spoon the mixture into the greased muffin cups evenly. Bake in the preheated oven for about 12 minutes, or until the tops spring back lightly when gently pressed with your fingertip.
6. Remove from the oven and allow to cool for about 6 minutes, then serve warm.

TIP: The almond meal can be substituted for the almond flour, and the texture is a little different.

PER SERVING
calories: 259 | fat: 23.3g | protein: 8.1g | net carbs: 4.1g | fiber: 2g

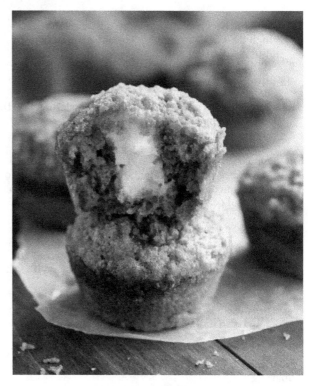

Ingredients:

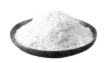

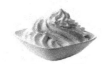

4 tablespoons melted butter, plus more for greasing the muffin tin

¾ tablespoon baking powder

1 cup almond flour

2 large eggs, lightly beaten

2 ounces (57 g) cream cheese mixed with 2 tablespoons heavy whipping cream

SPECIAL EQUIPMENT:

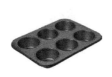
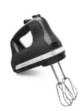

A 6-cup muffin tin   A hand mixer

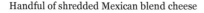

Handful of shredded Mexican blend cheese

BACON AND EGG AVOCADO BREAKFAST WRAP

Macros: Fat 77% | Protein 20% | Carbs 3%

Prep time: 10 minutes | Cook time: 10 minutes | Serves 2

1. Add the bacon slices to a large skillet over medium-high heat, and fry for 6 to 8 minutes until crispy, flipping occasionally.
2. With a slotted spoon, transfer the bacon to a paper towel-lined platter. Reserve the bacon grease in the skillet for later use.
3. Beat the eggs and heavy cream in a bowl, then add the salt and pepper. Stir well.
4. Slowly pour the egg mixture into the skillet with the reserved bacon grease, swirling the pan to spread evenly.
5. Cook for 1 minute, lifting the edges with a spatula to let the uncooked egg mixture flow underneath. Flip it over and cook for 1 minute more until set.
6. Fold one edge of the omelet over and slice in half, then transfer to two serving plates lined with paper towels, allowing the extra grease to soak up.
7. Make the wraps: Scatter each top with the cooked bacon, spinach, and avocado slices. Season with salt and pepper, then roll the wraps and serve.

TIP: Just use an extra egg instead of the heavy cream to make this dish dairy-free.

PER SERVING
calories: 341 | fat: 29.3g | protein: 17.2g | net carbs: 2.1g | fiber: 3g

Ingredients:

6 bacon slices

2 large eggs

2 tablespoons heavy whipping cream

1 cup fresh spinach, chopped

½ avocado, sliced

Pink Himalayan salt, to taste

Freshly ground black pepper, to taste

BLUEBERRY NUTTY OATMEAL

Macros: Fat 80% | Protein 16% | Carbs 4%

Prep time: 10 minutes | Cook time: 6 to 8 hours | Serves 6

1. Coat the insert of a slow cooker with melted coconut oil.
2. Put all ingredients except for the blueberries in the slow cooker, and stir until completely mixed.
3. Cook covered on LOW for about 6 to 8 hours.
4. Divide the oatmeal among six serving bowls and garnish with the blueberries before serving.

TIP: To add more flavors to this oatmeal, serve topped with a dollop of plain Greek yogurt.

PER SERVING
calories: 372 | fat: 33.2g | protein: 14.3g | net carbs: 3.9g | fiber: 6g | cholesterol: 0mg

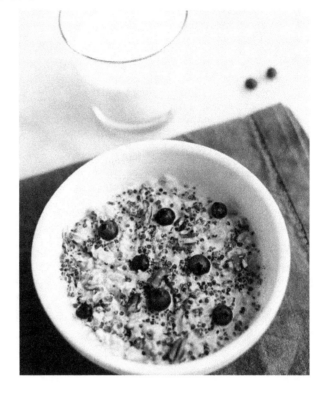

Ingredients:

1 tablespoon coconut oil, melted

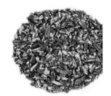

½ cup chopped pecans

½ cup sliced almonds

1 avocado, diced

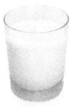

1 cup coconut milk

1 cup unsweetened coconut, shredded

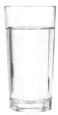

2 cups water

2 ounces (57 g) protein powder

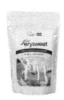

¼ cup granulated erythritol

1 teaspoon ground cinnamon

¼ teaspoon ground nutmeg

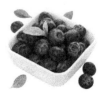

½ cup blueberries, for garnish

MUSHROOM AND SPINACH CHEESE FRITTATA

Macros: Fat 78% | Protein 20% | Carbs 2%

Prep time: 10 minutes | Cook time: 25 minutes | Serves 6

1. Preheat the oven to 350°F (180°C).
2. In a large ovenproof skillet, heat the olive oil over medium-high heat. Add the mushrooms and fry for 3 minutes until they start to brown, stirring frequently.
3. Fold in the bacon and spinach and cook for about 1 to 2 minutes, or until the spinach is wilted.
4. Slowly pour in the beaten eggs and cook for 3 to 4 minutes. Using a spatula to lift the edges for allowing uncooked egg to flow underneath.
5. Top with the goat cheese, then sprinkle the salt and pepper to season.
6. Bake in the preheated oven for about 15 minutes until lightly golden brown around the edges.
7. Transfer to a plate and allow to cool slightly before slicing into wedges.

TIP: If you don't like goat cheese, it can be replaced with feta cheese higher in fat.

PER SERVING
calories: 315 | fat: 27.3g | protein: 16.2g | net carbs: 1.1g | fiber: 0g

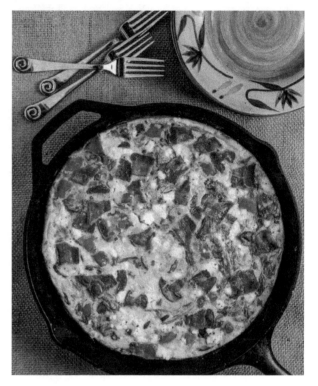

Ingredients:

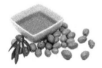

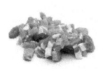

| 2 tablespoons olive oil | 1 cup fresh mushrooms, sliced | 6 bacon slices, cooked and chopped | 1 cup spinach, shredded | 10 large eggs, beaten | ½ cup goat cheese, crumbled |

Sea salt and freshly ground black pepper, to taste

KETO GOAT CHEESE SALMON FAT BOMBS

Macros: Fat 83% | Protein 17% | Carbs 0%

Prep time: 10 minutes | Cook time: 0 minutes | Makes 12 fat bombs

1. Line a baking sheet with parchment paper. Set aside.
2. Make the fat bombs: Mix the butter, goat cheese, smoked salmon, pepper, and lemon juice together in a bowl. Stir well to incorporate.
3. Scoop tablespoon-sized mounds of the mixture onto the parchment-lined baking sheet.
4. Transfer the fat bombs to the fridge for 2 to 3 hours until firm but not completely solid.
5. Remove from the fridge and let stand at room temperature for 8 minutes before serving.

TIP: Store the fat bombs in a sealed airtight container in the fridge for up to 1 week.

PER SERVING
calories: 196 | fat: 18.2g | protein: 8.1g | net carbs: 0g | fiber: 0g

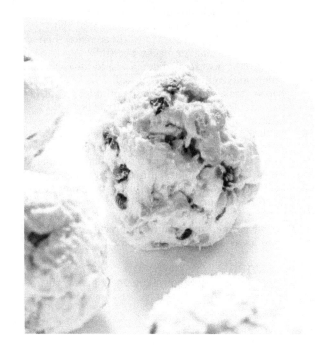

Ingredients:

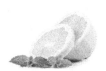

| ½ cup butter, at room temperature | ½ cup goat cheese, at room temperature | 2 ounces (57 g) smoked salmon | 2 teaspoons freshly squeezed lemon juice | Pinch freshly ground black pepper |

CAULIFLOWER BREAKFAST HASH

Macros: Fat 64% | Protein 26% | Carbs 10%

Prep time: 5 minutes | Cook time: 15 minutes | Serves 2

1. Add the bacon slices to a large skillet over medium-high heat, and cook for about 3 to 4 minutes on each side until evenly crisp.
2. Leave the bacon grease in the skillet and allow the bacon to cool on a paper towel-lined plate, then crumble into smaller pieces. Set aside.
3. Reduce the heat to medium, and add the garlic, onion, and cauliflower to the skillet with the bacon grease. Sauté for about 5 minutes or until the cauliflower starts to brown. If needed, add 1 tablespoon olive oil.
4. With the back of a spoon, make 4 evenly spaced wells in the cauliflower mixture, then crack an egg into each well. Sprinkle with the salt and pepper. Cook for 3 to 4 minutes, until the eggs are set.
5. Scatter the crumbled bacon pieces over the mixture and serve hot.

TIP: To save time, you can buy the precut vegetables, like cauliflower florets or broccoli florets.

PER SERVING
calories: 391 | fat: 27.3g | protein: 25.2g | net carbs: 10.2g | fiber: 4g

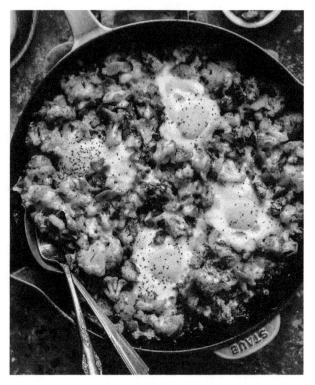

Ingredients:

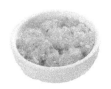

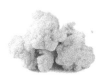

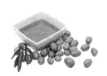

| 6 bacon slices | 2 minced garlic cloves | 1 diced medium onion | ½ head cauliflower, cut into small florets | 1 tablespoon olive oil, if needed | 4 large eggs |

Pink Himalayan salt, to taste

Freshly ground black pepper, to taste

CRAB SALAD STUFFED AVOCADOS

Macros: Fat 74% | Protein 20% | Carbs 6%

Prep time: 20 minutes | Cook time: 0 minutes | Serves 2

1. Make the crab salad: Place the cream cheese, crab meat, cucumber, red pepper, cilantro, scallion, salt, and pepper in a medium bowl. Mix well until blended. Set aside.
2. On a clean work surface, rub the cut parts of the avocado with fresh lemon juice.
3. Using a spoon, stuff each avocado halve with the crab salad. Serve immediately, or cover them with plastic wrap and refrigerate until ready to serve.

TIP: The crab salad can be made ahead and refrigerated until you want to stuff the avocado halves.

PER SERVING
calories: 378 | fat: 31.2g | protein: 19.2g | net carbs: 5.1g | fiber: 5g

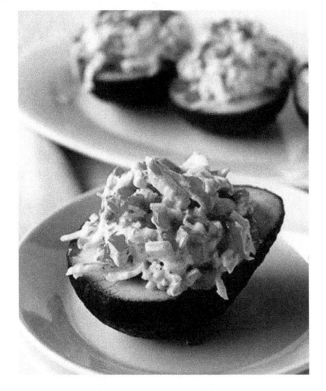

CRAB SALAD:

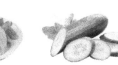
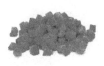

| ½ cup cream cheese | 4½ ounces (128 g) Dungeness crab meat | ¼ cup chopped, peeled English cucumber | ¼ cup chopped red bell pepper | 1 teaspoon chopped cilantro | ½ scallion, chopped |

STUFFED AVOCADOS:

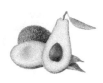
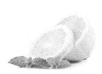

Pinch sea salt and freshly ground black pepper, to taste   1 avocado, peeled, halved lengthwise, and pitted   ½ teaspoon freshly squeezed lemon juice

LOW-CARB COCONUT BREAD

Macros: Fat 78% | Protein 19% | Carbs 3%

Prep time: 10 minutes | Cook time: 3 to 4 hours | Make 8 slices

1. Coat the bottom of a loaf pan with softened butter.
2. Mix together the beaten eggs, vanilla, coconut oil, and stevia in a bowl until combined well. Set aside.
3. Add the coconut flour, almond flour, baking powder, and protein powder in a separate bowl. Mix well.
4. Pour the dry ingredients into the bowl of wet ingredients, and stir well until a smooth batter forms.
5. Pour the batter into the prepared loaf pan on a rack in the slow cooker, and smooth the top with a spatula.
6. Cook covered on LOW until a sharp knife inserted in the center comes out clean, for about 3 to 4 hours.
7. Allow the bread to cool for about 10 minutes in the loaf pan, then transfer to a wire rack to cool completely before slicing.

TIP: If you are not keen on butter, coconut oil is an excellent alternative.

PER SERVING
calories: 327 | fat: 28.3g | protein: 15.2g | net carbs: 2.8g | fiber: 6g | cholesterol: 164mg

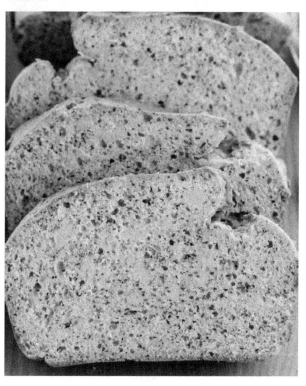

Ingredients:

1 tablespoon butter, softened

6 large eggs, lightly beaten

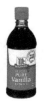

1 teaspoon pure vanilla extract

½ cup coconut oil, melted

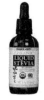

¼ teaspoon liquid stevia

½ cup coconut flour

SPECIAL EQUIPMENT:

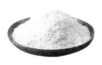

1 cup almond flour

1 teaspoon baking powder

1 ounce (28 g) protein powder

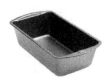

A loaf pan

FISH AND SEAFOOD

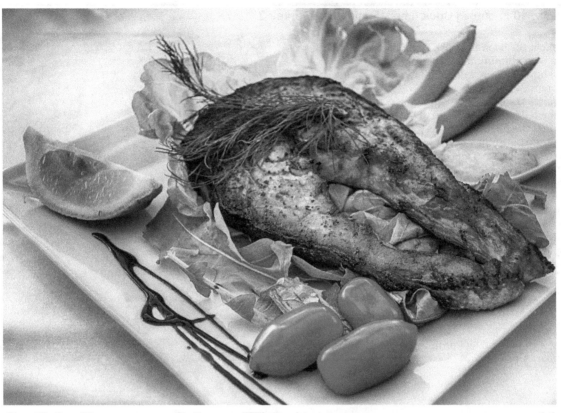

GARLICKY PARMESAN SALMON WITH ASPARAGUS

Macros: Fat 55% | Protein 39% | Carbs 6%

Prep time: 10 minutes | Cook time: 15 minutes | Serves 2

1. Preheat the oven to 400°F (205°C). Line a baking pan with aluminum foil and set aside.
2. In a bowl, rub the salmon fillets with salt and pepper.
3. Arrange the seasoned salmon fillets in the center of the baking pan and spread the asparagus around the fillets. Set aside.
4. Melt the butter in a skillet over medium heat. Toss in the garlic cloves and cook for about 3 minutes until fragrant, stirring constantly.
5. Pour the butter mixture over the salmon fillets and asparagus. Scatter the Parmesan cheese on top.
6. Bake in the preheated oven for 12 minutes, or until the fish flakes easily with a fork and the asparagus is fork-tender.
7. Remove from the oven and serve hot.

TIP: The asparagus can be replaced with fresh green beans.

PER SERVING
calories: 430 | fat: 26.3g | protein: 42.2g | net carbs: 6.2g | fiber: 5.1g

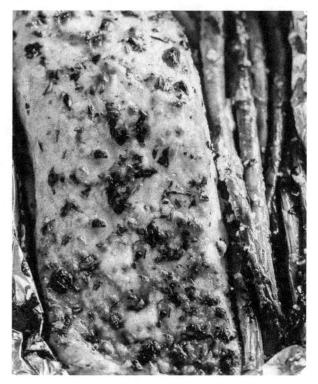

Ingredients:

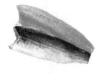

2 (6-ounce / 170-g) salmon fillets, skin on and patted dry

Pink Himalayan salt, to taste

Freshly ground black pepper, to taste

1 pound (454 g) fresh asparagus, ends snapped off

3 tablespoons butter

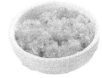

2 minced garlic cloves

¼ cup Parmesan cheese, shredded

FRIED PORK RIND CRUSTED SALMON CAKES

Macros: Fat 74% | Protein 25% | Carbs 1%

Prep time: 10 minutes | Cook time: 12 minutes | Serves 4

1. Mix together the salmon, beaten egg, pork rinds, 1½ tablespoons mayo, salt, and pepper in a large bowl until well combined.
2. Make the salmon cakes: On a lightly floured surface, scoop out 2 tablespoons of the salmon mixture and shape into a patty with your palm, about ½ inch thick. Repeat with the remaining salmon mixture.
3. Melt the ghee in a large skillet over medium-high heat. Fry the patties for about 6 minutes until golden brown on both sides, flipping once.
4. Remove from the heat to a plate lined with paper towels. Set aside.
5. Combine the remaining mayo and mustard in a small bowl. Stir well.
6. Serve the salmon cakes with the mayo dipping sauce on the side.

TIP: If you don't have a large skillet that fits all the patties, you can cook them in batches.

PER SERVING
calories: 382.9 | fat: 31.3g | protein: 24.2g | net carbs: 1.1g | fiber: 0g

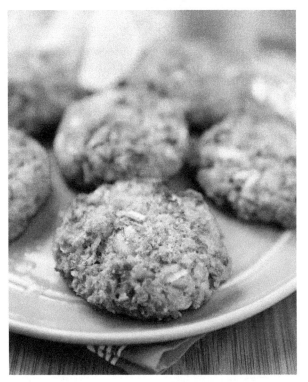

SALMON CAKES:

  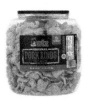

| 6 ounces (170 g) canned Alaska wild salmon, drained | 1 egg, lightly beaten | 2 tablespoons pork rinds, crushed | 3 tablespoons mayonnaise, divided | Pink Himalayan salt, to taste | Freshly ground black pepper, to taste1 |

MAYO DIPPING SAUCE:

1 tablespoon ghee   ½ tablespoon Dijon mustard

BAKED SALMON WITH MAYO SAUCE

Macros: Fat 72% | Protein 26% | Carbs 2%

Prep time: 10 minutes | Cook time: 10 minutes | Serves 2

1. Preheat the oven to 450°F (235°C). Generously grease a baking dish with melted ghee.
2. In a bowl, rub the salmon fillets with salt and pepper, then transfer to the greased baking dish.
3. Mix together the mayo, mustard, garlic powder, and dill in a small bowl. Brush both sides of each fillets generously with the mayo mixture.
4. Bake in the preheated oven for about 7 to 9 minutes until cooked through.
5. Remove from the oven and serve on plates.

TIP: You can bake your fish to desired doneness: medium, or well done, between 7 to 9 minutes.

PER SERVING
calories: 512.9 | fat: 41.3g | protein: 33.2g | net carbs: 2.1g | fiber: 1g

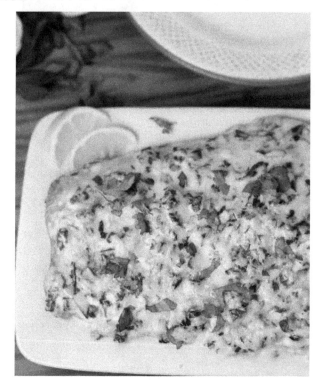

SALMON:

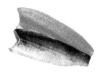

| 2 tablespoons ghee, melted | 2 (6-ounce) salmon fillets, skin on and patted dry | Pink Himalayan salt, to taste | Freshly ground black pepper, to taste |

MAYO SAUCE:

| ¼ cup mayonnaise | 1 tablespoon Dijon mustard | Pinch garlic powder | 2 tablespoons fresh dill, minced |

BUTTERED SCALLOPS WITH HERBS

Macros: Fat 70% | Protein 25% | Carbs 5%

Prep time: 10 minutes | Cook time: 10 minutes | Serves 4

1. In a bowl, lightly season the sea scallops with black pepper.
2. Melt 2 tablespoons butter in a large skillet over medium heat. Fry the scallops about 2 to 3 minutes on each side, or until golden brown.
3. Remove from the heat and set the sea scallops aside on a plate.
4. Melt the remaining butter in the same skillet and sauté the garlic about 3 minutes until tender.
5. Add the sea scallops, basil, thyme, and lemon juice, and cook for 2 minutes more.
6. Remove from the heat and serve on plates.

TIP: To add more flavors to this meal, you can serve garnished with chopped parsley.

PER SERVING
calories: 311.9 | fat: 24.3g | protein: 19.2g | net carbs: 4.1g | fiber: 0g

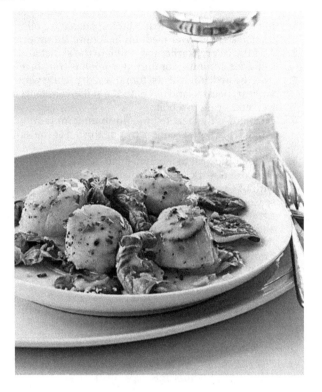

Ingredients:

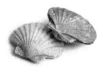

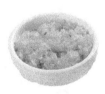

1 pound (454 g) sea scallops, cleaned and patted dry

Freshly ground black pepper, to taste

8 tablespoons butter, divided

2 teaspoons minced garlic

2 teaspoons chopped fresh basil

1 teaspoon chopped fresh thyme

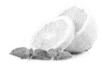

Juice of 1 lemon

ARTICHOKE CAPONATA WITH GRILLED SALMON FILLETS

Macros: Fat 67% | Protein 28% | Carbs 5%

Prep time: 15 minutes | Cook time: 20 minutes | Serves 4

1. Make the caponata: Heat 3 tablespoons olive oil in a nonstick skillet over medium heat until shimmering.
2. Add the celery, garlic, and onion to the skillet and sauté for 4 minutes or until the onion is translucent.
3. Add the artichoke heats, tomatoes, dry white wine, vinegar, pecans, and olives to the skillet. Sauté to mix well and bring to a boil.
4. Turn down the heat to low and simmer for 6 minutes or until the liquid reduces by one third. Set the skillet aside.
5. Preheat the grill to medium-high heat.
6. On a clean work surface, brush the salmon fillets with olive oil, and sprinkle the salt and pepper to season.
7. Arrange the salmon on the preheated grill grates, and grill for 8 minutes or until cooked through. Flip the salmon halfway through.
8. Transfer the salmon to four plates, and pour the caponata over each salmon and serve with basil on top.

TIP: To make it a complete meal, you can serve it with roasted green beans and spicy chicken stew.

PER SERVING
calories: 340.9 | fat: 25.3g | protein: 24.2g | net carbs: 4.1g | fiber: 3g | Sodium:128

CAPONATA:

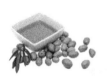	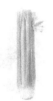				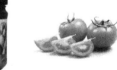
¼ cup olive oil, divided	2 celery stalks, chopped	1 tablespoon garlic, minced	1 onion, chopped	½ cup marinated artichoke hearts, chopped	2 tomatoes, chopped

2 tablespoons dry white wine	¼ cup apple cider vinegar	2 tablespoons chopped pecans	¼ cup pitted green olives, chopped	4 (4-ounce / 113-g) salmon fillets	Freshly ground black pepper, to taste	2 tablespoons chopped fresh basil, for garnish

LEMONY AND SPICY SHRIMP

Macros: Fat 56% | Protein 39% | Carbs 5%

Prep time: 10 minutes | Cook time: 15 minutes | Serves 2

1. Preheat the oven to 425°F (220°C).
2. Cut one half of lemon into slices, and cut another half of lemon into two wedges.
3. Put the melted butter on a baking dish, add the shrimp and garlic to the baking dish. Sprinkle the salt, black pepper, and red pepper flakes to season.
4. Add the lemon slices to the baking dish. Bake in the preheated oven for 15 minutes. Flip the shrimp halfway through the cooking time or until the shrimp is a little white in color.
5. Transfer the cooked shrimp to a large plate, and squeeze the lemon wedges on top before serving.

TIP: To make it a complete meal, you can serve it with garlicky roasted broccoli and creamy chicken soup.

PER SERVING
calories: 327.9 | fat: 20.3g | protein: 32.2g | net carbs: 4.1g | fiber: 1g

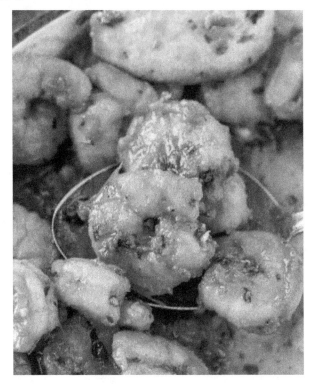

Ingredients:

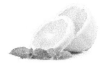

1 lemon, halved

3 tablespoons melted butter

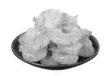

½ pound (227 g) shrimp, peeled and deveined, with tail off

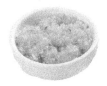

2 garlic cloves, crushed

¼ teaspoon red pepper flakes

Pink Himalayan salt and freshly ground black pepper, to taste

FRIED HALIBUT WITH CITRUS SAUCE

Macros: Fat 71% | Protein 26% | Carbs 3%

Prep time: 10 minutes | Cook time: 15 minutes | Serves 4

1. On a clean work surface, pat the halibut fillets dry with paper towels. Rub both sides of each fillet with salt and pepper, then set them aside on a plate.
2. In a saucepan, melt the butter over medium heat. Add the garlic and shallots, and sauté for about 3 minutes until fragrant.
3. Pour in the lemon juice, lime juice, and white wine while whisking. Bring the liquid to a simmer for 2 minutes until the citrus sauce is thickened.
4. Remove from the heat and scatter the parsley over the sauce. Set aside.
5. Heat the olive oil in a large skillet over medium-high heat. Add the seasoned fillets and fry for 5 minutes per side until lightly browned.
6. Remove the fillets from the heat to four serving plates and drizzle each fillet with the citrus sauce. Serve warm.

TIP: You can try any of your favourite fish, such as tilapia, sea bass or haddock.

PER SERVING
calories: 334.8 | fat: 26.4g | protein: 22.2g | net carbs: 2.1g | fiber: 0g

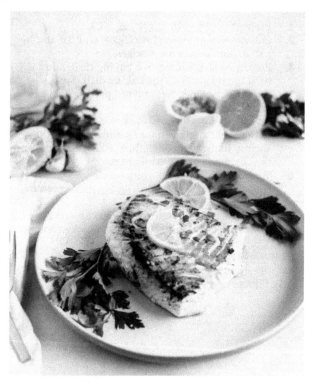

FISH:

   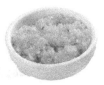 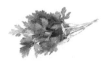

| 4 (5-ounce / 142-g) halibut fillets, each about 1 inch thick | Sea salt and freshly ground black pepper, to taste | 2 teaspoons garlic, minced | 1 minced shallot | 2 teaspoons fresh parsley, chopped |

CITRUS SAUCE:

 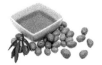 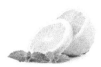 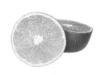

| ¼ cup butter | 2 tablespoons olive oil | 1 tablespoon freshly squeezed lemon juice | 1 tablespoon freshly squeezed lime juice | 3 tablespoons dry white wine |

FISH CURRY WITH KALE AND CILANTRO

Macros: Fat 70% | Protein 26% | Carbs 4%

Prep time: 10 minutes | Cook time: 20 minutes | Serves 4

1. In a large saucepan, melt the coconut oil over medium heat.
2. Add the garlic and ginger and sauté for about 2 minutes until tender.
3. Fold in the cumin and curry powder, then cook for 1 to 2 minutes until fragrant.
4. Add the coconut milk and bring it to a rapid boil. When it starts to boil, turn down the heat to low and allow to simmer until the flavors mellow, about 5 minutes.
5. Add the fish chunks and simmer for 10 minutes until the fish flakes easily with a fork, stirring once.
6. Scatter the shredded kale and chopped cilantro over the fish, then cook for 2 minutes more until softened.
7. Allow to cool for 5 minutes before serving.

TIP: The fish curry perfectly pairs with a bowl of cauliflower rice.

PER SERVING
calories: 402.9 | fat: 31.3g | protein: 26.2g | net carbs: 4.1g | fiber: 1g

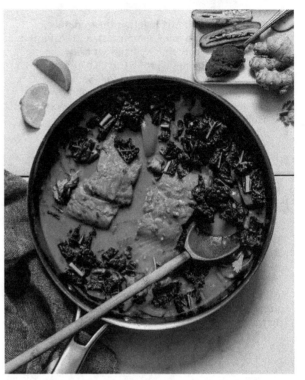

Ingredients:

2 tablespoons coconut oil

2 teaspoons garlic, minced

1½ tablespoons grated fresh ginger

½ teaspoon ground cumin

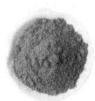

1 tablespoon curry powder

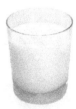

2 cups coconut milk

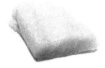

16 ounces (454 g) firm white fish, cut into 1-inch chunks

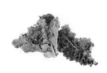

1 cup kale, shredded

2 tablespoons cilantro, chopped

BROWNED SALMON WITH TOMATO SALAD

Macros: Fat 72% | Protein 27% | Carbs 1%

Prep time: 15 minutes | Cook time: 15 minutes | Serves 4

1. Make the salad: Mix together the tomatoes, avocado, lemon juice, lemon zest, and scallion in a bowl. Stir to combine well and set aside.
2. Preheat the oven to 400°F (205°C) and line a baking sheet with aluminum foil. Set aside.
3. Combine the coriander, cumin, onion powder, cayenne, salt, and pepper in a separate bowl. Mix well.
4. Slather the fillets with the spice mixture, then transfer to the prepared baking sheet.
5. Pour the olive oil over each fillet and roast in the preheated oven for 15 minutes until just cooked through.
6. Remove the fish from the heat and serve alongside the tomato salad.

TIP: The salmon fillets can be cooked ahead of time, cooled completely, and cover with plastic wrap in the refrigerator until you make the salad.

PER SERVING
calories: 329.9 | fat: 26.3g | protein: 22.2g | net carbs: 1.1g | fiber: 3g

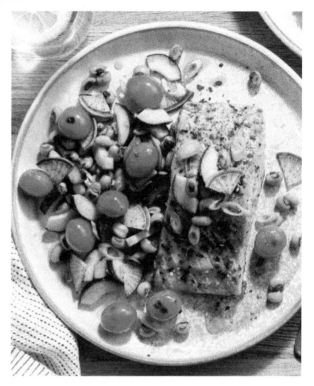

SALAD:

½ cup halved cherry tomatoes

1 avocado, peeled, pitted, and diced

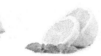
Juice of 1 lemon

Zest of 1 lemon

1 scallion, white and green parts, chopped

FISH:

½ teaspoon ground coriander

1 teaspoon ground cumin

½ teaspoon onion powder

Pinch cayenne pepper

¼ teaspoon sea salt

Pinch freshly ground black pepper

4 (4-ounce / 113-g) boneless, skinless salmon fillets

2 tablespoons olive oil

CRISPY PROSCIUTTO-WRAPPED HADDOCK FILLETS

Macros: Fat 57% | Protein 40% | Carbs 3%

Prep time: 10 minutes | Cook time: 17 minutes | Serves 4

1. Preheat the oven to 350°F (180°C) and line a baking sheet with parchment paper. Set aside.
2. In a bowl, lightly season the haddock fillets with salt and pepper. Tightly wrap each fillet with a slice of prosciutto.
3. Arrange the prosciutto-wrapped fillets on the prepared baking sheet and drizzle with olive oil.
4. Bake in the preheated oven until cooked through, about 15 to 17 minutes.
5. Serve topped with the lemon juice and zest.

TIP: Don't rip the prosciutto slices while preparing the fish.

PER SERVING
calories: 285.9 | fat: 18.3g | protein: 29.2g | net carbs: 1.1g | fiber: 0g | Sodium:76mg

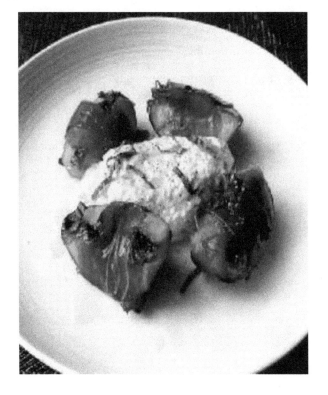

Ingredients:

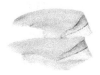

4 (4-ounce / 113-g) haddock fillets, about 1 inch thick, patted dry

Sea salt and freshly ground black pepper, to taste

4 slices (2-ounce / 57-g) prosciutto

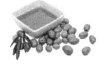

3 tablespoons olive oil

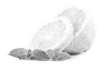

Juice and zest of 1 lemon

CHEESY AND BUTTERED SALMON

Macros: Fat 70% | Protein 27% | Carbs 3%

Prep time: 15 minutes | Cook time: 12 minutes | Serves 4

1. Preheat the oven to 350°F (180°C) and line a baking sheet with parchment paper. Set aside.
2. Make the topping: Combine the butter, Asiago cheese, garlic, lemon juice, basil, and oregano in a bowl. Toss well until completely mixed.
3. Arrange the salmon fillets, skin-side down, on the prepared baking sheet. Divide the topping among the fillets and with the back of a spoon, spread it all over. Pour the olive oil over the fillets.
4. Bake in the preheated oven for about 12 minutes, or until the topping is golden brown and the fish flakes easily with a fork.
5. Remove from the oven and serve hot.

TIP: Store the salmon fillets in a sealed airtight container in the fridge for 4 days or in the freezer for up to one month.

PER SERVING
calories: 359.9 | fat: 28.3g | protein: 24.2g | net carbs: 2.1g | fiber: 0g

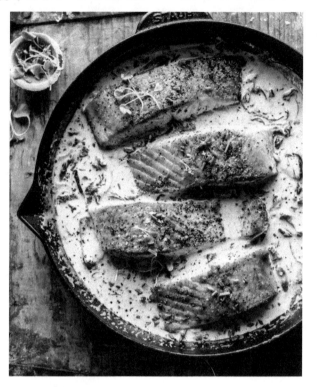

TOPPING:

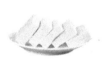   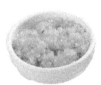 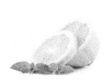

| 2 tablespoons butter, at room temperature | ½ cup Asiago cheese | 2 teaspoons minced garlic | 2 tablespoons freshly squeezed lemon juice | 1 teaspoon chopped fresh basil | 1 teaspoon chopped fresh oregano |

FISH:

4 (5-ounce / 142-g) salmon fillets, patted dry   1 tablespoon olive oil

SALAD

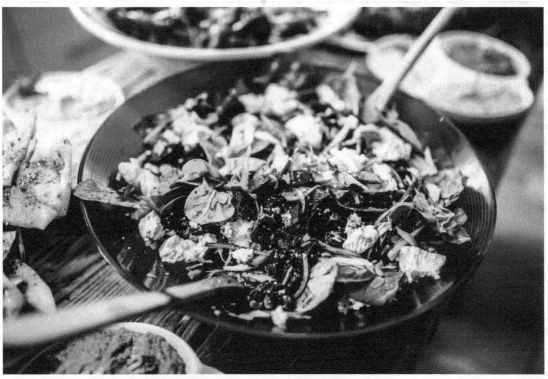

KALE SALAD WITH THE BACON AND BLUE CHEESE

Macros: Fat 74% | Protein 18% | Carbs 8%

Prep time: 10 minutes | Cook time: 10 minutes | Serves 2

1. Add the bacon slices to a skillet over medium-high heat, and fry for 3 to 4 minutes on each side until evenly crisp.
2. With a slotted spoon, transfer the bacon to a plate lined with paper towels. Set aside to cool.
3. In a large bowl, pour the vinaigrette over the kale and massage it into the kale with your hands. Season with salt and pepper, then allow to stand for 5 minutes.
4. Make the salad: Chop the cooked bacon and pecans on you cutting board. Transfer them to the bowl of kale, and top with a sprinkle of blue cheese. Toss the mixture until well blended.
5. To serve , divide the salad between two serving plates.

TIP: The chopped almond can be substituted for the chopped pecans in this recipe.

PER SERVING
calories: 356.9 | fat: 29.3g | protein: 16.2g | net carbs: 7.1g | fiber: 3g

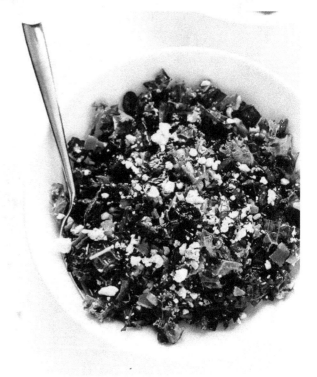

Ingredients:

4 bacon slices

1 tablespoon vinaigrette salad dressing

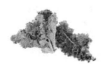

2 cups fresh kale, stemmed and chopped

Pinch pink Himalayan salt

Pinch freshly ground black pepper

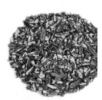

¼ cup pecans

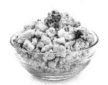

¼ cup crumbled blue cheese

GREEK SALAD WITH VINAIGRETTE SALAD DRESSING

Macros: Fat 85% | Protein 8% | Carbs 7%

Prep time: 10 minutes | Cook time: 0 minutes | Serves 2

1. Make the salad: Stir together the tomatoes, romaine lettuce, feta cheese, olives, and vinaigrette in a large bowl.
2. Sprinkle with salt and pepper, then pour over the olive oil. Toss the salad until well combined.
3. To serve, divide the salad between two serving bowls.

TIP: If you want to add additional flavor and freshness, you can mix in the chopped cucumbers or red onion.

PER SERVING
calories: 202.9 | fat: 19.3g | protein: 4.2g | net carbs: 3.1g | fiber: 2g

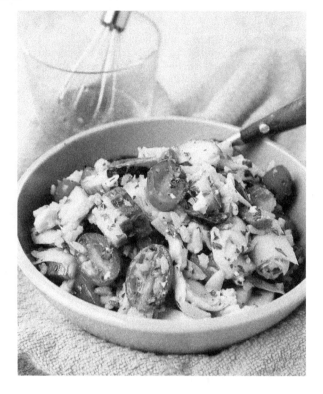

Ingredients:

½ cup halved grape tomatoes

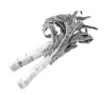

2 cups chopped romaine lettuce

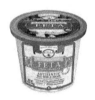

¼ cup feta cheese crumbles

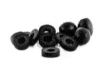

¼ cup sliced black olives

2 tablespoons vinaigrette salad dressing

Pink Himalayan salt, to taste

Freshly ground black pepper, to taste

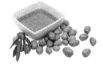

1 tablespoon olive oil

BACON AVOCADO SALAD

Macros: Fat 87% | Protein 8% | Carbs 5%

Prep time: 20 minutes | Cook time: 0 minutes | Serves 4

1. In a large bowl, mix together the eggs, spinach, avocados, lettuce, and onion. Set aside.
2. Make the vinaigrette: In a separate bowl, add the olive oil, mustard, and apple cider vinegar. Mix well.
3. Pour the vinaigrette into the large bowl and toss well.
4. Serve topped with bacon slices and sliced avocado.

TIP:To add more flavors to this meal, serve with a sprinkle of Parmesan cheese.

PER SERVING
calories: 342.5 | fat: 33.3g | protein: 7.2g | net carbs: 3.5g

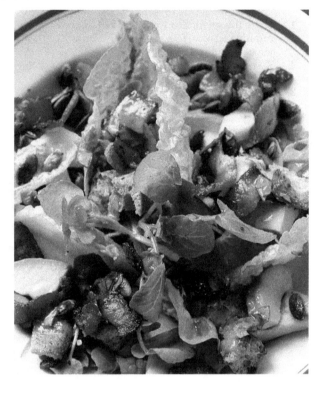

Ingredients:

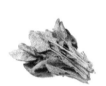

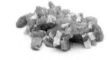

| 2 hard-boiled eggs, chopped | 2 cups spinach | 2 large avocados, 1 chopped and 1 sliced | 2 small lettuce heads, chopped | 1 spring onion, sliced | 4 cooked bacon slices, crumbled |

VINAIGRETTE

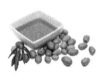

| 3 tablespoons olive oil | 1 teaspoon Dijon mustard | 1 tablespoon apple cider vinegar |

CAULIFLOWER, SHRIMP AND CUCUMBER SALAD

Macros: Fat 66% | Protein 27% | Carbs 7%

Prep time: 10 minutes | Cook time: 15 minutes | Serves 6

1. In a skillet over medium heat, heat the olive oil until sizzling hot. Add the shrimp and cook for 8 minutes, stirring occasionally, or until the flesh is totally pink and opaque.
2. Meanwhile, in a microwave-safe bowl, add the cauliflower florets and microwave for about 5 minutes until tender.
3. Remove the shrimp from the heat to a large bowl. Add the cauliflower and cucumber to the shrimp in the bowl. Set aside.
4. Make the dressing: Mix together the olive oil, lemon juice, lemon zest, dill, salt, and pepper in a third bowl. Pour the dressing into the bowl of shrimp mixture. Toss well until the shrimp and vegetables are coated thoroughly.
5. Serve immediately or refrigerate for 1 hour before serving.

TIP: The shrimp can be cooked ahead of time, cooled completely, and cover with plastic wrap in the refrigerator until you make the salad.

PER SERVING
calories: 236.9 | fat: 17.3g | protein: 15.2g | net carbs: 5.1g

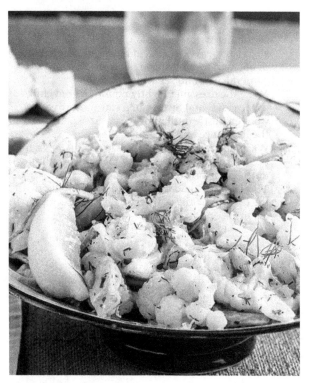

Ingredients:

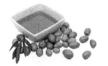

¼ cup olive oil

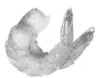

1 pound (454 g) medium shrimp

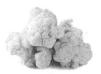

1 cauliflower head, florets only

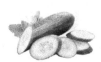

2 cucumber, peeled and chopped

DRESSING

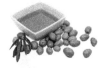

1 tablespoon olive oil

¼ cup lemon juice

2 tablespoons lemon zest

3 tablespoons dill, chopped

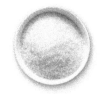

Salt and pepper, to taste

SEARED SQUID SALAD WITH RED CHILI DRESSING

Macros: Fat 66% | Protein 28% | Carbs 6%

Prep time: 20 minutes | Cook time: 5 minutes | Serves 4

1. Make the salad: Mix together the arugula, cucumber strips, red onion, mint leaves, and coriander leaves in a salad bowl. Add the salt, pepper, and 1 tablespoon olive oil. Toss to combine well and set aside.
2. Make the dressing: Lightly pound the red chili, garlic clove, and Swerve in a clay mortar with a wooden pestle until it forms a coarse paste. Mix in the lime juice and fish sauce. Set aside.
3. Warm the remaining olive oil in a skillet over high heat. Add the squid and sear for about 5 minutes until lightly browned.
4. Transfer the squid to the salad bowl and top with the dressing. Stir well. Serve garnished with the cilantro.

TIP: For a unique twist, you can make this salad with beef besides squid.

PER SERVING
calories: 332.5 | fat: 24.5g | protein: 23.5g | net carbs: 4.5g

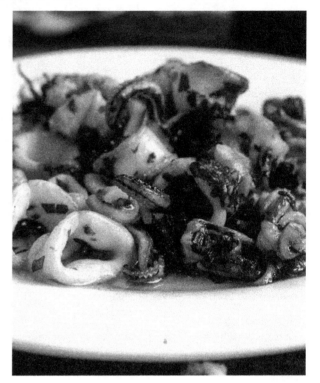

Ingredients:

SALAD:

| 4 medium squid tubes, cut into rings | 1 tablespoon chopped cilantro, for garnish | 1 cup arugula | 2 medium cucumbers, halved and cut in strips | ½ red onion, finely sliced | ½ cup mint leaves | ½ cup cilantro leaves, reserve the stems |

DRESSING:

| Salt and black pepper, to taste | 2 tablespoons olive oil, divided | 1 red chili, roughly chopped | 1 clove garlic | 1 teaspoon Swerve | 2 limes, juiced | 1 teaspoon fish sauce |

CAULIFLOWER AND CASHEW NUT SALAD

Macros: Fat 77% | Protein 13% | Carbs 10%

Prep time: 10 minutes | Cook time: 5 minutes | Serves 4

1. Add the cauliflower into a pot of boiling salted water. Allow to boil for 4 to 5 minutes until fork-tender but still crisp.
2. Remove from the heat and drain on paper towels, then transfer the cauliflower to a bowl.
3. Add the olives, bell pepper, and red onion. Stir well.
4. Make the dressing: In a separate bowl, mix together the olive oil, mustard, vinegar, salt, and pepper. Pour the dressing over the veggies and toss to combine.
5. Serve topped with cashew nuts and celery leaves.

TIP: Blanching the cauliflower can give it a desired and uniform texture.

PER SERVING
calories: 196.7 | fat: 16.3g | protein: 6.3g | net carbs: 6.2g

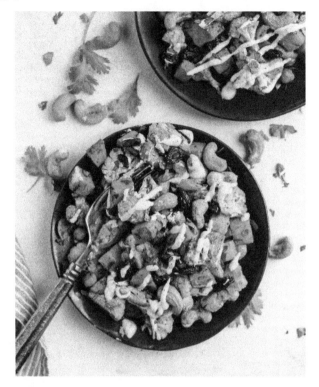

Ingredients:

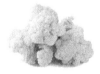

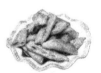

| 1 head cauliflower, cut into florets | ½ cup black olives, pitted and chopped | 1 cup roasted bell peppers, chopped | 1 red onion, sliced | ½ cup cashew nuts | Chopped celery leaves, for garnish |

DRESSING:

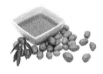

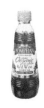

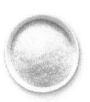

| ¼ cup extra-virgin olive oil | 1 teaspoon yellow mustard | 1 tablespoon wine vinegar | Salt and black pepper, to taste | |

SALMON AND LETTUCE SALAD

Macros: Fat 80% | Protein 15% | Carbs 5%

Prep time: 10 minutes | Cook time: 0 minutes | Serves 4

1. In a bowl, stir together the olive oil, salmon, mayo, lime juice, and salt. Stir well until the salmon is coated fully.
2. Divide evenly the romaine lettuce and onion flakes among four serving plates. Spread the salmon mixture over the lettuce, then serve topped with avocado slices.

TIP: The taste of avocado slices will be much stronger if you refrigerate the salad for 30 minutes before serving.

PER SERVING
calories: 227.1 | fat: 20.3g | protein: 8.8g | net carbs: 2.3g

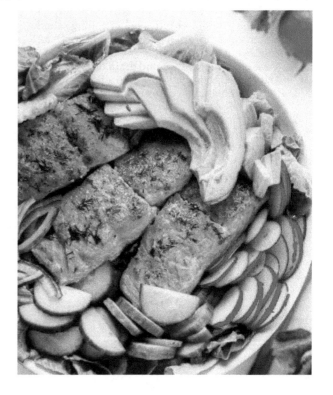

Ingredients:

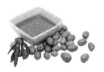   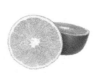 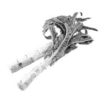

| 1 tablespoon extra virgin olive oil | 2 slices smoked salmon, chopped | 3 tablespoons mayonnaise | 1 tablespoon lime juice | Sea salt, to taste | 1 cup romaine lettuce, shredded |

1 teaspoon onion flakes   ½ avocado, sliced

PRAWNS SALAD WITH MIXED LETTUCE GREENS

Macros: Fat 84% | Protein 12% | Carbs 4%

Prep time: 10 minutes | Cook time: 3 minutes | Serves 4

1. In a bowl, add the prawns, salt, and chili pepper. Toss well.
2. Warm the olive oil over medium heat. Add the seasoned prawns and fry for about 6 to 8 minutes, stirring occasionally, or until the prawns are opaque.
3. Remove from the heat and set the prawns aside on a platter.
4. Make the dressing: In a small bowl, mix together the mustard, aioli, and lemon juice until creamy and smooth.
5. Make the salad: In a separate bowl, add the mixed lettuce greens. Pour the dressing over the greens and toss to combine.
6. Divide the salad among four serving plates and serve it alongside the prawns.

TIP: The prawns can be done ahead, cooled completely, and cover with plastic wrap in the refrigerator until you serve the salad.

PER SERVING
calories: 226.9 | fat: 21.3g | protein: 6.9g | net carbs: 1.9g

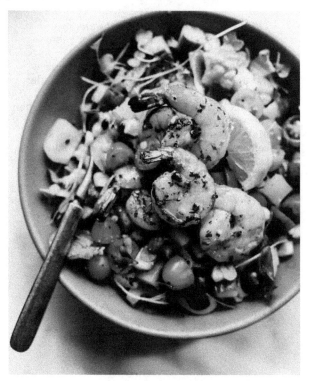

Ingredients:

DRESSING:

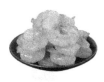

½ pound (227 g) prawns, peeled and deveined

Salt and chili pepper, to taste

1 tablespoon olive oil

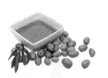

2 cups mixed lettuce greens

½ teaspoon Dijon mustard

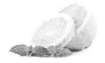

1 tablespoon lemon juice

¼ cup aioli

POACHED EGG SALAD WITH LETTUCE AND OLIVES

Macros: Fat 67% | Protein 24% | Carbs 9%

Prep time: 10 minutes | Cook time: 10 minutes | Serves 4

1. Put the eggs into a pot of salted water over medium heat, then bring to a boil for about 8 minutes.
2. Using a slotted spoon, remove the eggs one at a time from the hot water. Let them cool under running cold water in the sink. When cooled, peel the eggs and slice into bite-sized pieces, then transfer to a large bowl.
3. Make the salad: Add the romaine lettuce, stalk celery, mayo, mustard, sriracha sauce, lime juice, salt, and pepper to the bowl of egg pieces . Toss to combine well.
4. Evenly divide the salad among four serving plates. Serve garnished with scallions and sliced black olives.

TIP: You can store the salad in a sealed airtight container in the fridge for up to 2 to 3 days. It is not recommended to freeze.

PER SERVING
calories: 291.8 | fat: 21.8g | protein: 17.7g | net carbs: 6.2g

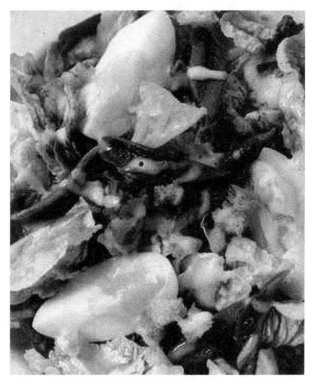

Ingredients:

4 eggs

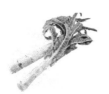

1 head romaine lettuce, torn into pieces

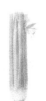

¼ stalk celery, minced

¼ cup mayonnaise

½ tablespoon mustard

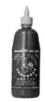

½ teaspoon low-carb sriracha sauce

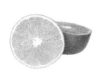

¼ teaspoon fresh lime juice

Salt and black pepper, to taste

¼ cup chopped scallions, for garnish

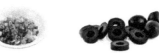

10 sliced black olives, for garnish

BEEF SALAD WITH VEGETABLES

Macros: Fat 58% | Protein 35% | Carbs 7%

Prep time: 10 minutes | Cook time: 10 minutes | Serves 4

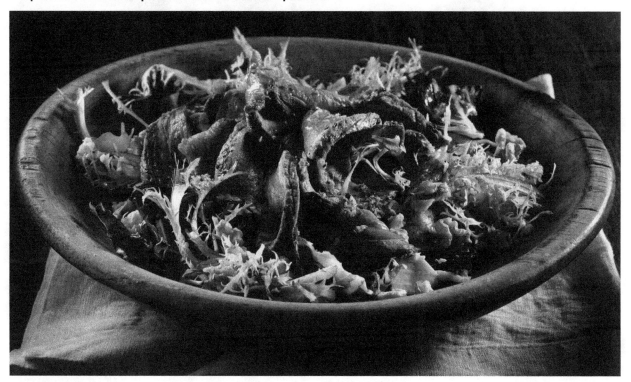

MEATABALLS:

1 pound (454 g) ground beef

¼ cup pork rinds, crushed

1 egg, whisked

1 onion, grated

1 tablespoon fresh parsley, chopped

½ teaspoon dried oregano

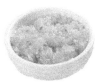

1 garlic clove, minced

Salt and black pepper, to taste

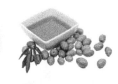

2 tablespoons olive oil, divided

SALAD:

1 cup chopped
arugula

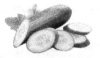

1 cucumber, sliced

1 cup cherry
tomatoes, halved

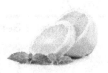

1½ tablespoons
lemon juice

Salt and pepper, to taste

DRESSING:

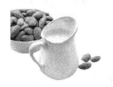

2 tablespoons
almond milk

1 cup plain Greek
yogurt

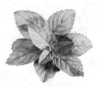

1 tablespoon fresh
mint, chopped

1. Stir together the beef, pork rinds, whisked egg, onion, parsley, oregano, garlic, salt, and pepper in a large bowl until completely mixed.
2. Make the meatballs: On a lightly floured surface, using a cookie scoop to scoop out equal-sized amounts of the beef mixture and form into meatballs with your palm.
3. Heat 1 tablespoon olive oil in a large skillet over medium heat, fry the meatballs for about 4 minutes on each side until cooked through.
4. Remove from the heat and set aside on a plate to cool.
5. In a salad bowl, mix together the arugula, cucumber, cherry tomatoes, 1 tablespoon olive oil, and lemon juice. Season with salt and pepper.
6. Make the dressing: In a third bowl, whisk the almond milk, yogurt, and mint until well blended. Pour the mixture over the salad. Serve topped with the meatballs.

TIP: If you don't have a large skillet that fits all the meatballs, you can cook them in batches.

PER SERVING
calories: 487.2 | fat: 31.6g | protein: 42.2g | net carbs: 8.5g

NIÇOISE SALAD

Macros: Fat 76% | Protein 19% | Carbs 5%

Prep time: 5 minutes | Cook time: 30 minutes | Serves 6

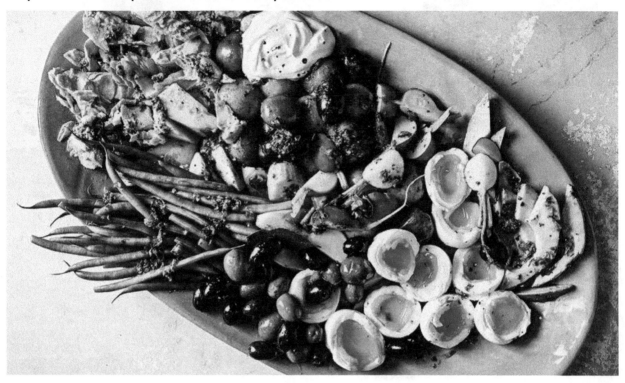

DRESSING:

¾ cup MCT oil

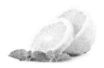

½ cup lemon juice

1 teaspoon Dijon mustard

1 tablespoon fresh thyme leaves, minced

1 medium shallot, minced

2 teaspoons fresh oregano leaves, minced

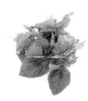

2 tablespoons fresh basil leaves, minced

Celtic sea salt and freshly ground black pepper, to taste

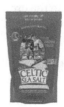

SALAD:

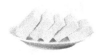

2 tablespoons butter

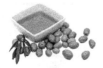

1 tablespoon olive oil

2 (8-ounce / 227-g) tuna steaks

2 heads of red leaf lettuce, washed and torn into bite-sized pieces

8 ounces (227 g) green beans, stem ends trimmed and each bean halved crosswise

6 hard-boiled eggs, peeled and quartered

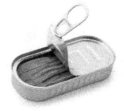

1 can anchovies, or more as needed

1 avocado, peeled and sliced into chunks

¼ cup olives

3 small tomatoes, sliced

1. Melt the butter and heat the olive oil in a nonstick skillet over medium-high heat. Place the tuna steaks in the skillet, and sear for 3 minutes or until opaque, flipping once. Set aside.
2. Make the dressing: Combine all the ingredients for the dressing in a bowl.
3. Make six niçoise salads: Dunk the lettuce and tuna steaks in the dressing bowl to coat well, then arrange the tuna in the middle of the lettuce. Set aside.
4. Blanch the green beans in a pot of boiling salted water for 3 to 5 minutes or until soft but still crisp. Drain and dry with paper towels.
5. Dunk the green beans in the dressing bowl to coat well. Arrange them around the tuna steaks on the lettuce.
6. Top the tuna and green beans with hard-boiled eggs, anchovies, avocado chunks, tomatoes, and olives. Sprinkle 2 tablespoons dressing over the each egg, then serve.

TIP: To make this a complete meal, you can top it with grilled rib eye steak or serve it with salmon soup and roasted duck.

PER SERVING
calories: 502 | total fat: 42.2g | carbs: 8.8g | protein: 23.6g

SHRIMP, TOMATO, AND AVOCADO SALAD

Macros: Fat 65% | Protein 29% | Carbs 6%

Prep time: 5 minutes | Cook time: 30 minutes | Serves 4

1. Combine the shrimp, tomatoes, avocados, cilantro, and onions in a large bowl.
2. Squeeze the lemon juice over the vegetables in the large bowl, then drizzle with avocado oil and sprinkle the salt and black pepper to season. Toss to combine well.
3. You can cover the salad, and refrigerate to chill for 45 minutes or serve immediately.

TIP: To make this a complete meal, you can top it with grilled rib eye steak or serve it with chicken soup and roasted turkey.

PER SERVING
calories: 382 | total fat: 27.2g | carbs: 5.8g | protein: 28.1g

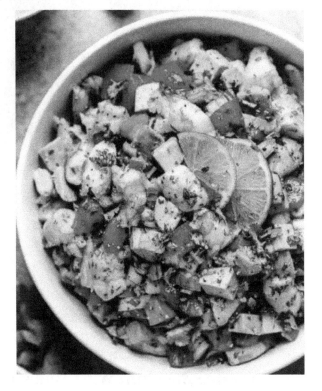

Ingredients:

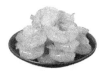

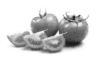

1 pound (454 g) shrimp, shelled and deveined

2 tomatoes, cubed

2 avocados, peeled and cubed

A handful of fresh cilantro, chopped

4 green onions, minced

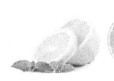

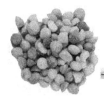

Juice of 1 lime or lemon

1 tablespoon macadamia nut or avocado oil

Celtic sea salt and fresh ground black pepper, to taste

VEGETABLE

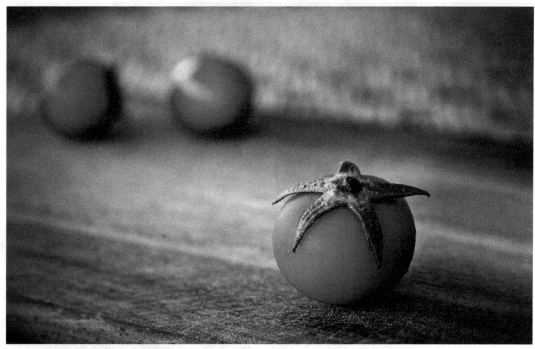

SIMPLE SAUTÉED ASPARAGUS SPEARS WITH WALNUTS

Macros: Fat 84% | Protein 10% | Carbs 6%

Prep time: 10 minutes | Cook time: 5 minutes | Serves 4

1. In a large skillet over medium-high heat, heat the olive oil.
2. Add the asparagus and sauté for about 5 minutes until fork-tender, stirring occasionally.
3. Sprinkle with salt and pepper, then transfer to a large bowl.
4. Serve topped with chopped walnuts.

TIP: Blanching the asparagus can give it a smoother texture and an irresistible flavor.

PER SERVING
calories: 131.9 | fat: 12.3g | protein: 3.2g | net carbs: 2.1g | fiber: 2g

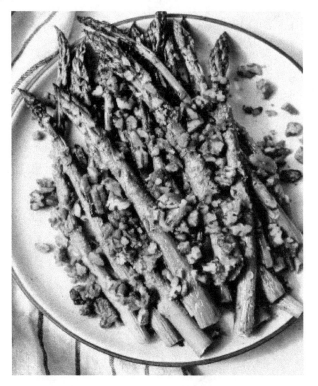

Ingredients:

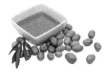
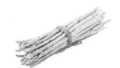

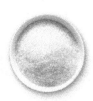

| 1½ tablespoons olive oil | ¾ pound (340 g) asparagus spears, woody ends trimmed | Sea salt and freshly ground pepper, to taste | ¼ cup walnuts, chopped |

CAULIFLOWER MASH

Macros: Fat 72% | Protein 18% | Carbs 10%

Prep time: 15 minutes | Cook time: 5 minutes | Serves 4

1. Fill a large saucepan three-quarters full with water and bring the water to a boil over high heat
2. Blanch the cauliflower in the boiling water for about 4 to 5 minutes, until it starts to soften.
3. Remove from the heat and drain on a paper towel.
4. Put the cauliflower to a food processor, along with the heavy cream, cheese, and butter. Process until it's creamy and fluffy. Sprinkle with the salt and pepper.
5. Divide the cauliflower mixture among four serving bowls, and serve.

TIP: The cauliflower mash perfectly goes well with baked coconut chicken.

PER SERVING
calories: 193.7 | fat: 15.3g | protein: 8.2g | net carbs: 5.8g | fiber: 2g

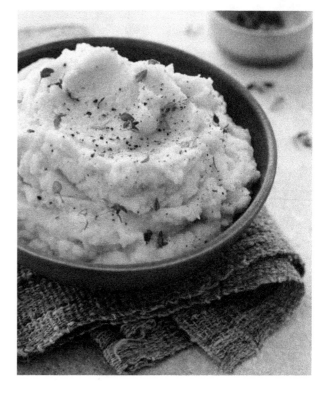

Ingredients:

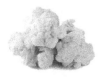   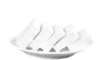

| 1 head cauliflower, chopped roughly | ¼ cup heavy whipping cream | ½ cup shredded Cheddar cheese | 2 tablespoons butter, at room temperature | Sea salt and freshly ground black pepper, to taste |

TENDER ZUCCHINI WITH CHEESE

Macros: Fat 78% | Protein 17% | Carbs 5%

Prep time: 15 minutes | Cook time: 10 minutes | Serves 4

1. Melt the butter in a large frying pan over medium-high heat.
2. Sauté the zucchini in the melted butter for about 5 minutes, stirring frequently, or until the zucchini is tender but still crisp.
3. Scatter the grated Parmesan cheese over the zucchini. Cook for 5 minutes more until the cheese melts. Season as desired with salt and pepper.
4. Remove from the heat and serve on plates.

TIP: To add more flavors to this meal, garnish it with fresh basil or a handful of chopped chives.

PER SERVING
calories: 95.9 | fat: 8.3g | protein: 4.2g | net carbs: 1.1g | fiber: 0g

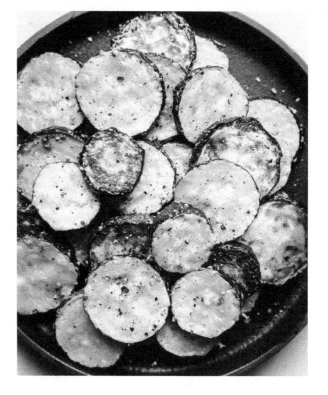

Ingredients:

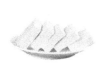

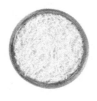

2 tablespoons butter   4 zucchini, cut into ¼-inch-thick rounds   ½ cup freshly grated Parmesan cheese   Freshly ground black pepper, to taste

VEGGIE CHILI WITH AVOCADO CREAM

Macros: Fat 87% | Protein 6% | Carbs 7%

Prep time: 10 minutes | Cook time: 25 minutes | Serves 8

1. In a large skillet, warm the olive oil over medium-high heat.
2. Toss in the onion, garlic, jalapeño peppers, and red bell pepper, then sauté for about for 4 minutes until tender. Add the cumin and chili powder, and stir for 30 seconds.
3. Fold in the pecans, tomatoes and their juice, then bring to a boil. Reduce the heat to low and allow to simmer uncovered for about 20 minutes to infuse the flavors, stirring occasionally.
4. Remove from the heat to eight bowls. Evenly top each bowl of chili with the sour cream, diced avocado, and fresh cilantro.

TIP: To add more flavors to this meal, serve topped with a sprinkle of Cheddar cheese.

PER SERVING
calories: 332.3 | fat: 32.3g | protein: 5.3g | net carbs: 5.1g | fiber: 6g | Sodium: 194mg

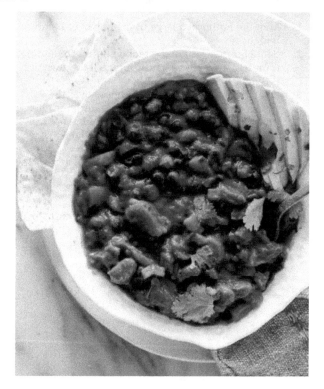

Ingredients:

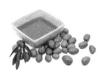

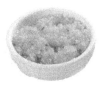

| 2 tablespoons olive oil | ½ onion, finely chopped | 1 tablespoon minced garlic | 2 jalapeño peppers, chopped | 1 red bell pepper, diced | 1 teaspoon ground cumin |

TOPPING:

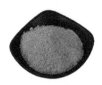

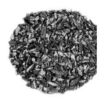

| 2 tablespoons chili powder | 2 cups pecans, chopped | 4 cups canned diced tomatoes and their juice | 1 cup sour cream | 1 avocado, diced | 2 tablespoons fresh cilantro, chopped |

SLOW COOKER CREAMED VEGETABLES

Macros: Fat 78% | Protein 15% | Carbs 7%

Prep time: 15 minutes | Cook time: 6 hours | Serves 6

1. Coat the insert of a slow cooker with olive oil.
2. Put the remaining ingredients in the greased slow cooker, then stir to combine.
3. Cook covered on LOW for about 6 hours, or until the vegetables are tender.
4. Remove from the heat and serve warm.

TIP: You can try any of your favorite vegetables, such as bok choy, Brussels sprouts, and broccoli.

PER SERVING
calories: 209.9 | fat: 18.3g | protein: 8.2g | net carbs: 3.1g | fiber: 2g | cholesterol: 42mg

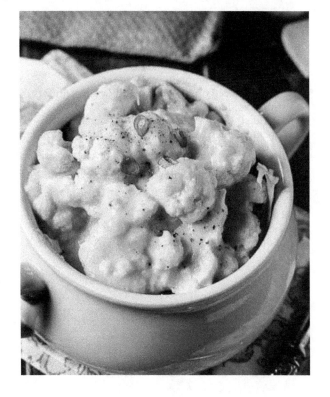

Ingredients:

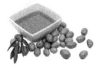

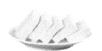

1 tablespoon extra-virgin olive oil	3 tablespoons butter	2 cups green beans, cut into 2-inch pieces	1 cup asparagus spears, cut into 2-inch pieces	½ head cauliflower, cut into small florets	½ cup sour cream

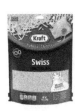

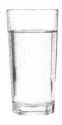

½ cup shredded Cheddar cheese	½ cup shredded swiss cheese	¼ cup water	1 teaspoon ground nutmeg	Pinch freshly ground black pepper

CAULIFLOWER AN PECAN CASSEROLE WITH PECANS

Macros: Fat 74% | Protein 20% | Carbs 6%

Prep time: 5 minutes | Cook time: 6 hours | Serves 6

1. Coat the insert of a slow cooker with olive oil.
2. Combine the cauliflower, pecans, bacon, salt, garlic, and pepper in a medium bowl. Toss well.
3. Transfer to the slow cooker and drizzle the mixture with lemon juice.
4. Cook covered on LOW for about 6 hours until the top is golden brown.
5. Divide the casserole among six serving bowls. Sprinkle the shredded eggs and scallion on top for garnish before serving.

TIP: You can store the leftovers in an airtight container in the fridge for up to 4 days.

PER SERVING
calories: 282.9 | fat: 23.3g | protein: 14.2g | net carbs: 4.1g | fiber: 5g |cholesterol: 123mg

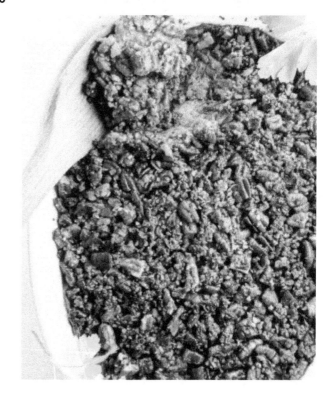

Ingredients:

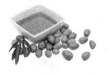

1 tablespoon extra-virgin olive oil

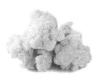

2 pounds (907 g) cauliflower florets

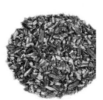

1 cup chopped pecans

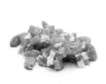

10 bacon slices, cooked and chopped

4 garlic cloves, sliced

½ teaspoon salt

½ teaspoon freshly ground black pepper

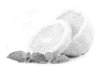

2 tablespoons freshly squeezed lemon juice

4 shredded hard-boiled eggs, for garnish

1 chopped scallion, for garnish

SWEET AND BUTTERY RED CABBAGE

Macros: Fat 71% | Protein 19% | Carbs 10%

Prep time: 15 minutes | Cook time: 7 to 8 hours | Serves 8

1. Coat the insert of a slow cooker with olive oil.
2. Put the cabbage, garlic, onion, cloves, apple cider vinegar, nutmeg, and erythritol in the slow cooker. Stir the mixture until completely mixed.
3. Drizzle the top with the melted butter, then cook covered on LOW for 7 to 8 hours until cooked through.
4. Add the salt and pepper. Stir well.
5. Remove from the slow cooker to serving bowls.
6. To serve, garnish with the walnuts, blue cheese, and pink peppercorns, if desired.

TIP: Don't shred or grate the red cabbage too finely, and using a food processor can save your time.

PER SERVING
calories: 155 | fat: 12.4g | protein: 7.3g | net carbs: 3.8g | fiber: 1g | cholesterol: 13mg

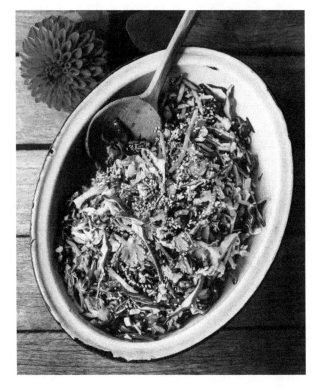

Ingredients:

1 tablespoon extra-virgin olive oil

1 small red cabbage, coarsely shredded (about 6 cups)

2 teaspoons minced garlic

½ sweet onion, thinly sliced

⅛ teaspoon ground cloves

¼ cup apple cider vinegar

½ teaspoon ground nutmeg

3 tablespoons granulated erythritol

2 tablespoons butter, melted

Salt and freshly ground black pepper, to taste

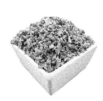

½ cup chopped walnuts, for garnish

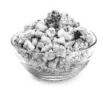

½ cup blue cheese crumbles, for garnish

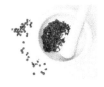

Pinch Pink peppercorns, for garnish (optional)

CHEESY KALE STUFFED ZUCCHINI

Macros: Fat 76% | Protein 19% | Carbs 5%

Prep time: 10 minutes | Cook time: 30 minutes | Serves 2

1. Preheat the oven to 375°F (190°C). Coat a baking sheet with 1 tablespoon olive oil.
2. Spoon the zucchini pulp out, and reserve on a plate. Arrange the hollowed zucchini halves on the baking sheet.
3. Melt the butter in a nonstick skillet over medium heat, then sauté the garlic in the skillet for 4 minutes or until golden brown.
4. Add the reserved zucchini pulp and kale to the skillet and cook until the kale has wilted. Sprinkle the salt and black pepper to season.
5. Drizzle 2 tablespoons olive oil in the zucchini halves. Spread the zucchini pulp mixture in the zucchini halves, then scatter with Mozzarella cheese.
6. Place the baking sheet in the preheated oven and bake for 25 minutes or until the cheese melts.
7. Transfer the cooked zucchini to a large plate. Drizzle with olive oil, and sprinkle with salt and black pepper before serving.

TIP: To make this a complete meal, you can serve it with roasted chicken breasts and salmon soup.

PER SERVING
calories: 443 | total fat: 37.5g | carbs: 5.9g | protein: 20.5g

Ingredients:

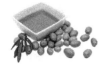

3 tablespoons olive oil, divided, plus more for topping

1 zucchini, halved

4 tablespoons butter

2 garlic cloves, minced

1½ ounces (680 g) baby kale

1 cup Mozzarella cheese, shredded

Salt and freshly ground black pepper, to taste

CHERRY TOMATO GRATIN

Macros: Fat 82% | Protein 11% | Carbs 7%

Prep time: 5 minutes | Cook time: 20 minutes | Serves 4

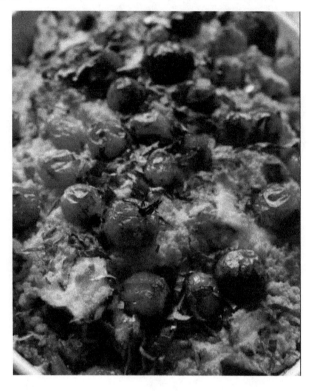

1. Preheat the oven to 350°F (180°C). Grease a baking pan with olive oil.
2. Combine the cherry tomatoes, mayo, vegan Mozzarella cheese, ½ ounce (14 g) of Parmesan cheese, basil pesto, salt, and black pepper in the baking pan.
3. Smooth the top with a spatula, then scatter with the remaining Parmesan. Bake in the preheated oven for 20 minutes or until lightly browned.
4. Remove them from the oven and divide among four plates. Top with watercress and olive oil, and slice to serve.

TIP: To make this a complete meal, you can serve it with roasted beef, or chicken and mushroom soup.

PER SERVING
calories: 451 | total fat: 41.2g | carbs: 4.7g | protein: 12.1g

Ingredients:

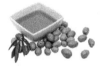

2 tablespoons olive oil, plus more for topping

½ cup cherry tomatoes, halved

½ cup mayonnaise, keto-friendly

½ cup vegan Mozzarella cheese, cut into pieces

1 ounce (28 g) vegan Parmesan cheese, shredded

1 tablespoon basil pesto

Salt and freshly ground black pepper, to taste

1 cup watercress

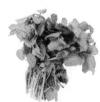

YOGURT, CHEESE, AND DILL STUFFED TOMATO

Macros: Fat 75% | Protein 18% | Carbs 7%

Prep time: 5 minutes | Cook time: 30 minutes | Serves 2

1. Preheat the oven to 400°F (205°C). Grease a baking sheet with olive oil.
2. Cut the tops of the tomatoes off, then spoon the tomato seeds and pulp out and reserve on a plate. Keep the tomato tops. Arrange the hollowed tomatoes on the baking sheet.
3. Whisk together the remaining ingredients, tomato seeds and pulp in a bowl.
4. Spoon the mixture into the hollowed tomatoes, then cover with the tomato tops.
5. Bake in the preheated oven for 30 minutes or until the tomatoes are lightly wilted. Transfer the cooked stuffed tomatoes to two plates. Allow to cool for 5 minutes before serving.

TIP: To make this a complete meal, you can top the stuffed tomatoes with fresh rocket leaves and serve it with pork chops, or chicken and mushroom soup.

PER SERVING
calories: 282 | total fat: 23.6g | carbs: 4.9g | protein: 12.4g

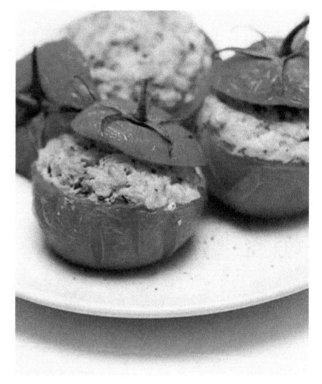

Ingredients:

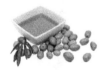

1 tablespoon olive oil

2 tomatoes

1 egg

Salt and freshly ground black pepper, to taste

1 clove garlic, minced

¼ cup Greek yogurt

¼ cup feta cheese, crumbled

2 tablespoons fresh dill, chopped

2 tablespoons butter, softened

BEEF, LAMB, AND PORK

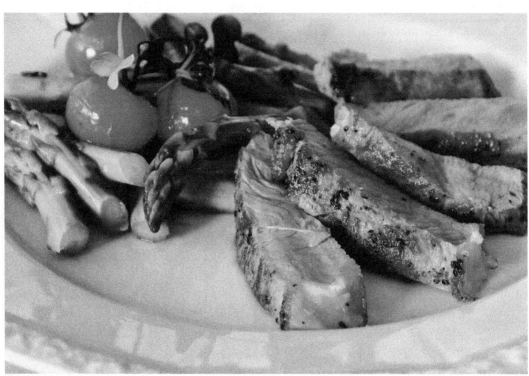

JERK PORK

Macros: Fat 72% | Protein 24% | Carbs 4%

Prep time: 15 minutes | Cook time: 20 minutes | Serves 6

1. Combine the ingredients for the seasoning in a bowl. Stir to mix well.
2. Put the pork rounds in the bowl of seasoning mixture. Toss to coat well.
3. Pour the olive oil in a nonstick skillet, and heat over medium-high heat.
4. Arrange the pork in the singer layer in the skillet and fry for 20 minutes or until an instant-read thermometer inserted in the center of the pork registers at least 145°F (63°C). Flip the pork rounds halfway through the cooking time. You may need to work in batches to avoid overcrowding.
5. Transfer the pork rounds onto a large platter, and top with cilantro and sour cream, then serve warm.

TIP: To make this a complete meal, serve it with Brussels sprouts with Balsamic sauce. They also taste great paired with arugula salad.

PER SERVING
calories: 289 | total fat: 23.2g | total carbs: 2.8g | fiber: 0.9g | net carbs: 1.9g | protein: 17.2g

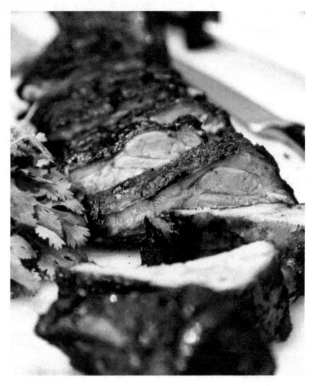

JERK SEASONING:

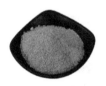

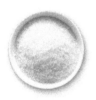

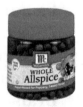

| ⅛ teaspoon cayenne pepper | ¼ teaspoon salt | ¼ teaspoon freshly ground black pepper | ½ tablespoon dried thyme | ½ tablespoon garlic powder | ½ tablespoon ground allspice |

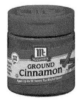

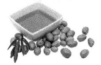

| 1 teaspoon ground cinnamon | 1 tablespoon granulated erythritol | 1 (1-pound / 454-g) pork tenderloin, cut into 1-inch rounds | ¼ cup extra-virgin olive oil | 2 tablespoons chopped fresh cilantro, for garnish | ½ cup sour cream |

HOT PORK AND BELL PEPPER IN LETTUCE

Macros: Fat 73% | Protein 21% | Carbs 6%

Prep time: 15 minutes | Cook time: 20 minutes | Serves 4

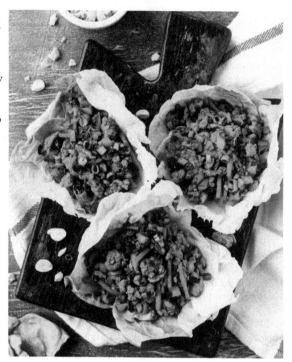

1. Make the sauce: Combine the ingredients for the sauce in a bowl. Set aside until ready to use.
2. Make the pork filling: In a nonstick skillet, warm a tablespoon sesame oil over medium-high heat.
3. Add the sauté the ground pork for 8 minutes or until lightly browned, then pour the sauce over and keep cooking for 4 minutes more or until the sauce has lightly thickened.
4. Transfer the pork onto a platter and set aside until ready to use.
5. Clean the skillet with paper towels, then warm the remaining sesame oil over medium-high heat.
6. Add and sauté the ginger and garlic for 3 minutes or until fragrant.
7. Add and sauté the sliced bell pepper and scallion for an additional 5 minutes or until fork-tender.
8. Lower the heat, and move the pork back to the skillet. Stir to combine well.
9. Divide and arrange the pork filling over four lettuce leaves and serve hot.

TIP: To make this a complete meal, serve it with Brussels sprouts with Balsamic sauce. They also taste great paired with arugula salad.

PER SERVING
calories: 385 | total fat: 31.1g | total carbs: 5.8g | fiber: 1.9g | net carbs: 3.9g | protein: 20.1g

SAUCE:

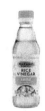
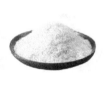
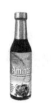

| 1 tablespoon fish sauce | 1 tablespoon rice vinegar | 1 tablespoon almond flour | 1 teaspoon coconut aminos | 1 tablespoon granulated erythritol | 2 tablespoons coconut oil |

PORK FILLING:

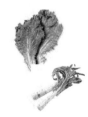

| 2 tablespoons sesame oil, divided | 1 pound (454 g) ground pork | 1 teaspoon fresh ginger, peeled and grated | 1 teaspoon garlic, minced | 1 red bell pepper, deseeded and thinly sliced | 1 scallion, white and green parts, thinly sliced | 8 large romaine or Boston lettuce leaves |

SAUSAGE, ZUCCHINI, EGGPLANT, AND TOMATO RATATOUILLE

Macros: Fat 70% | Protein 20% | Carbs 10%

Prep time: 15 minutes | Cook time: 45 minutes | Serves 4

1. Add the olive oil in a stock pot, and warm over medium-high heat, then add and sauté the Italian sausage meat for 7 minutes or until lightly browned.
2. Add the zucchini, bell pepper, eggplant, garlic, and onion to the pot and sauté for 10 minutes or until tender.
3. Fold in the balsamic vinegar, tomatoes, basil, and red pepper flakes. Stir to combine well, then bring to a boil.
4. Turn down the heat to low. Simmer the mixture for 25 minutes or until the vegetables are entirely softened.
5. Sprinkle with oregano, salt, and black pepper. Stir to mix well, then serve warm.

TIP: If you prefer the flavor of cheese or you want to enrich this recipe, you can scatter this ratatouille with shredded goat cheese or Mozzarella cheese and cook for another 2 or 3 minutes until the cheese melts, and you can also top it with a fried egg for more flavor.

PER SERVING
calories: 431 | total fat: 33.2g | total carbs: 11.8g | fiber: 4.2g | net carbs: 7.6g | protein: 21.2g

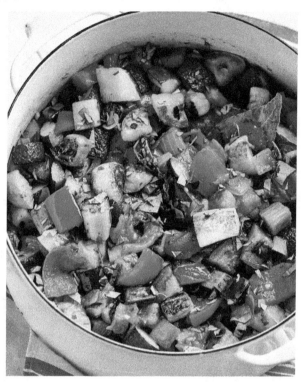

Ingredients:

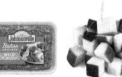

3 tablespoons extra-virgin olive oil	1 pound (454 g) Italian sausage meat (sweet or hot)	2 zucchini, diced	1 red bell pepper, diced	½ eggplant, cut into ½-inch cubes	1 tablespoon garlic, minced

½ red onion, chopped

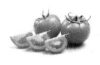

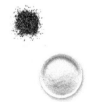

1 tablespoon balsamic vinegar

1 (15-ounce / 425-g) can low-sodium tomatoes, diced

1 tablespoon fresh basil, chopped

Red pepper flakes, to taste

2 teaspoons chopped fresh oregano, for garnish

Salt and freshly ground black pepper, to taste

BACON, BEEF, AND PECAN PATTIES

Macros: Fat 75% | Protein 23% | Carbs 2%

Prep time: 10 minutes | Cook time: 15 minutes | Serves 8

1. Preheat the oven to 450°F (235°C). Line a baking sheet with parchment paper.
2. Whisk together all the ingredients, except for the olive oil, in a bowl.
3. Grease your hands with olive oil, and shape the mixture into 8 patties with your hands.
4. Arrange the patties on the baking sheet and bake in the preheated oven for 20 minutes or until a meat thermometer inserted in the center of the patties reads at least 165°F (74°C). Flip the patties halfway through the cooking time.
5. Remove the cooked patties from the oven and serve warm.

TIP: You can serve the patties with the homemade sauces or store-bought burger toppings for more and different flavor.

PER SERVING
calories: 318 | total fat: 27.2g | total carbs: 1.1g | fiber: 1.1g | net carbs: 0g | protein: 18.1g

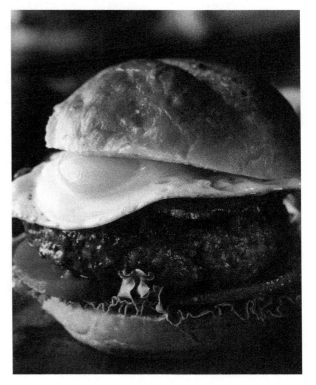

Ingredients:

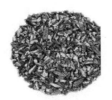

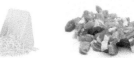

| ¼ cup chopped onion | ¼ cup ground pecans | 1 large egg | 2 ounces (57 g) Cheddar cheese, diced | 8 ounces (227 g) bacon, chopped | 1 pound (454 g) grass-fed ground beef |

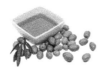

| Salt and freshly ground black pepper, to taste | 1 tablespoon extra-virgin olive oil |

LEMONY ANCHOVY BUTTER WITH STEAKS

Macros: Fat 76% | Protein 24% | Carbs 0%

Prep time: 15 minutes | Cook time: 10 minutes | Serves 4

1. Make the anchovy butter: Combine the anchovies, lemon juice, butter, and garlic in a bowl. Stir to mix well, then arrange the bowl into the refrigerator to chill until ready to use.
2. Preheat the grill to medium-high heat.
3. Rub the steaks with salt and black pepper on a clean work surface.
4. Arrange the seasoned steaks on the grill grates and grill for 10 minutes or until medium-rare. Flip the steaks halfway through the cooking time.
5. Allow the steaks to cool for 10 minutes. Transfer the steaks onto four plates, and spread the anchovy butter on top, then serve warm.

TIP: To make this a complete meal, you can serve it with spicy asparagus. They also taste great paired with fresh cucumber salad.

PER SERVING
calories: 447 | total fat: 38.1g | total carbs: 0g | fiber: 0g | net carbs: 0g | protein: 26.1g

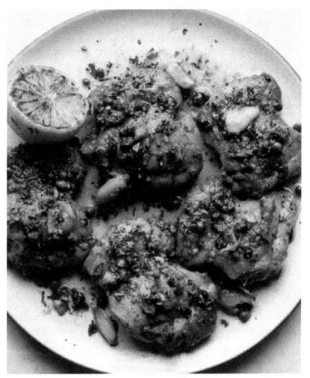

ANCHOVY BUTTER:

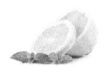

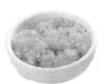

4 anchovies packed in oil, drained and minced

½ teaspoon freshly squeezed lemon juice

¼ cup unsalted butter, at room temperature

1 teaspoon minced garlic

4 (4-ounce / 113-g) rib eye steaks

Salt and freshly ground black pepper, to taste

ZUCCHINI CARBONARA

Macros: Fat 71% | Protein 23% | Carbs 6%

Prep time: 10 minutes | Cook time: 15 minutes | Serves 6

1. In a nonstick skillet, cook the bacon for 6 minutes or until it curls and buckle. Flip the bacon halfway through the cooking time.
2. Meanwhile, whisk together the eggs, egg yolks, ¼ cup of Parmesan cheese, cream, basil, parsley, salt, and black pepper in a large bowl. Set aside.
3. Add the garlic to the skillet and sauté for 3 minutes until fragrant, then pour the dry white wine over and cook for an additional 2 minutes for deglazing.
4. Turn down the heat to low, add and sauté the spiralized zucchini for 2 minutes.
5. Pour the egg mixture into the skillet and toss for 4 minutes or until the mixture is thickened and coat the spiralized zucchini.
6. Transfer to a platter and top with remaining cheese before serving.

TIP: To make this a complete meal, you can serve it with lemony radicchio salad. They alsao taste great paired with braised fennel and shallots.

PER SERVING
calories: 332 | total fat: 26.2g | total carbs: 6.9g | fiber: 2.1g | net carbs: 4.8g | protein: 19.1g

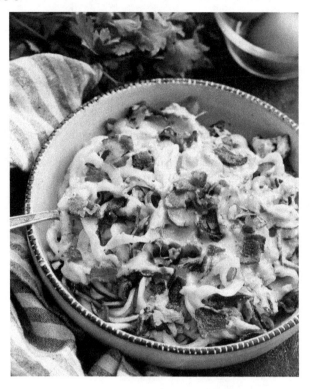

Ingredients:

8 chopped bacon slices

2 large eggs

4 large egg yolks

½ cup grated Parmesan cheese, divided

½ cup heavy whipping cream

2 tablespoons chopped fresh basil

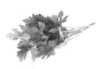

2 tablespoons chopped fresh parsley

Salt and freshly ground black pepper, to taste

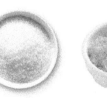

1 tablespoon minced garlic

½ cup dry white wine

4 medium zucchini, spiralized

MUSHROOM, SPINACH, AND ONION STUFFED MEATLOAF

Macros: Fat 72% | Protein 24% | Carbs 4%

Prep time: 20 minutes | Cook time: 1 hour | Serves 8

1. Preheat the oven to 350°F (180°C). Coat a meatloaf pan with olive oil.
2. Combine 1 pound (454 g) ground beef, cumin, garlic, salt, and black pepper in a large bowl. Pour the mixture into the meatloaf pan.
3. Make a well in the center of the beef mixture, then scatter the cheese on the bottom of the well. Put the mushrooms, spinach, and onions in the well, then cover them with the remaining 1 ounce (28 g) ground beef.
4. Place the meatloaf pan into the preheated oven and bake for 1 hour until cooked through.
5. Remove the meatloaf from the oven and slice to serve.

TIP: To gift this dish with more flavor. You can serve it with the homemade spicy or sour sauces, or store-bought toppings.

PER SERVING
calories: 254 | total fat: 20.2g | carbs: 1.4g | protein: 15.3g

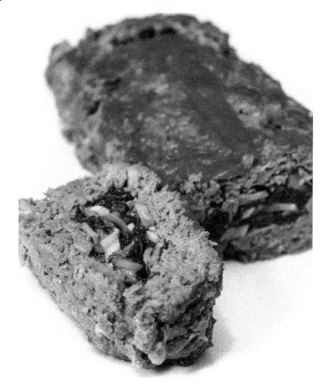

Ingredients:

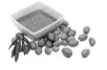

3 tablespoons extra-virgin olive oil

17 ounces (482 g) ground beef

2 teaspoons ground cumin

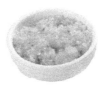

2 garlic cloves, granulated

Salt and freshly ground black pepper, to taste

6 slices Cheddar cheese

¼ cup mushrooms, diced

½ cup spinach

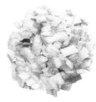

¼ cup onions, diced

¼ cup green onions, diced

ITALIAN FLAVOR HERBED PORK CHOPS

Macros: Fat 63% | Protein 37% | Carbs 0%

Prep time: 10 minutes | Cook time: 20 minutes | Serves 4

1. Preheat the oven to 350°F (180°C). Grease a baking dish with melted butter.
2. Combine the Italian seasoning, butter, olive oil, salt, and black pepper in a large bowl. Dredge each pork chop into the bowl to coat well.
3. Arrange the pork chops onto the baking dish, and spread the fresh parsley on top of each chop.
4. Bake in the preheated oven for 20 minutes or until cooked through. An instant-read thermometer inserted in the middle of the pork chops should register at least 145°F (63°C).
5. Transfer the pork chops from the oven and serve warm.

TIP: To make this a complete meal, you can serve it with roasted broccoli. They also taste great paired with creamy spinach and dill.

PER SERVING
calories: 335 | total fat: 23.4g | carbs: 0g | protein: 30.9g

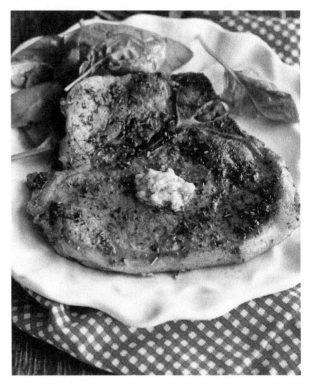

Ingredients:

2 tablespoons melted butter, plus more for coating

2 tablespoons Italian seasoning

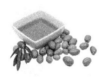

2 tablespoons olive oil

Salt and freshly ground black pepper, to taste (if no salt or pepper in the Italian seasoning)

4 pork chops, boneless

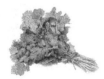

2 tablespoons fresh Italian leaf parsley, chopped

BRAISED BEEF SHANKS AND DRY RED WINE

Macros: Fat 32% | Protein 63% | Carbs 5%

Prep time: 10 minutes | Cook time: 8 hours | Serves 6

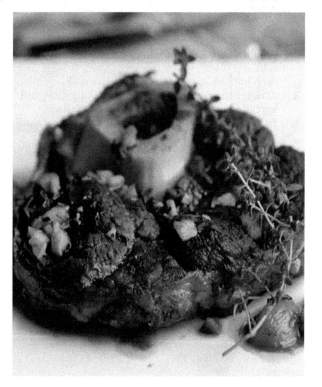

1. In a nonstick skillet, warm the olive oil over medium-high heat.
2. Put the beef shanks into the skillet and fry for 5 to 10 minutes until well browned. Flip the beef shanks halfway through. Set aside.
3. Pour the dry red wine into the skillet and bring to a simmer.
4. Coat the insert of the slow cooker with olive oil.
5. Add the cooked beef shanks, dry red wine, beef stock, rosemary, garlic, onion, salt, and black pepper to the slow cooker. Stir to mix well.
6. Put the slow cooker lid on and cook on LOW for 8 hours until the beef shanks are fork-tender.
7. Remove from the slow cooker and serve hot.

TIP: To make this a complete meal, you can serve it with roasted cauliflower. They also taste great paired with tomato and herb salad.

PER SERVING
calories: 315 | total fat: 11g | carbs: 4g | protein: 50g

Ingredients:

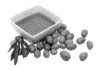

2 tablespoons olive oil

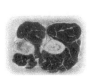

2 pounds (907 g) beef shanks

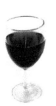

2 cups dry red wine

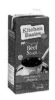

3 cups beef stock

1 sprig of fresh rosemary

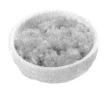

5 garlic cloves, finely chopped

1 onion, finely chopped

Salt and freshly ground black pepper, to taste

BEEF, EGGPLANT, ZUCCHINI, AND BABY SPINACH LASAGNA

Macros: Fat 50% | Protein 41% | Carbs 9%

Prep time: 10 minutes | Cook time: 4 hours | Serves 8

1. Warm the olive oil in a nonstick skillet over medium-high heat.
2. Add and sauté the garlic and onions for 3 minutes or until the onions are translucent.
3. Add and sauté the beef for 3 more minutes until lightly browned.
4. Add the dried mixed herbs and tomatoes over the beef, and season with salt and black pepper. Sauté for 5 minutes to combine well.
5. Grease the slow cooker with olive oil.
6. Make the lasagna: Spread a layer of beef mixture on the bottom of the slow cooker, and top the beef mixture with a layer of eggplant slices, then spread another layer of beef mixture, and then put on a layer of zucchini slices, after that, top the zucchini slices with a layer of beef mixture, and on the beef mixture, spread a layer of baby spinach leaves, and finally, a layer of beef mixture.
7. Combine all the cheeses, salt, and black pepper in a large bowl. Scatter the cheese mixture over the lasagna.
8. Put the slow cooker lid on and bake on HIGH for 4 hours.
9. Remove the hot lasagna from the slow cooker and slice to serve.

TIP: You can use different vegetables slices to replace the eggplant, zucchinis, or baby spinach leaves, such as tomato slices and broccoli slices.

PER SERVING
calories: 397 | total fat: 22.0g | carbs: 10.5g | protein: 40.8g

Ingredients:

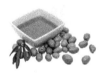
3 tablespoons olive oil, plus more for greasing the slow cooker

5 garlic cloves, finely chopped

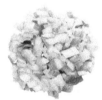
1 onion, finely chopped

2 pounds (907 g) beef, minced

2 teaspoons dried mixed herbs (oregano, rosemary, thyme)

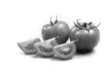
4 tomatoes, chopped

Salt and freshly ground black pepper, to taste

1 large eggplant, cut into round slices crosswise

2 large zucchinis, cut into slices lengthwise

2 cups baby spinach leaves

1 cup ricotta cheese

1 cup Mozzarella cheese, grated

2 cups Cheddar cheese, grated

LAMB AND TOMATO CURRY

Macros: Fat 60% | Protein 31% | Carbs 9%

Prep time: 10 minutes | Cook time: 8 hours | Serves 8

1. Warm the olive oil in a nonstick skillet over medium-high heat.
2. Add and sear the lamb shoulder for 3 minutes until browned on both sides.
3. Grease the slow cooker with olive oil.
4. Place the cooked lamb into the slow cooker, and add the curry paste, garlic, onions, salt, and black pepper. Toss to coat the lamb well.
5. Add the stock cube, tomatoes, coconut milk, and water to the slow cooker. Stir to mix well.
6. Put the slow cooker lid on and cook on LOW for 8 hours.
7. Transfer the lamb curry to a large plate, and spread the coriander and yogurt on top to serve.

TIP: To make this a complete meal, you can serve it with Indian raita, cucumber salad, and naan.

PER SERVING
calories: 406 | total fat: 28.2g | total carbs: 10.5g | fiber: 4.3g | net carbs: 6.2g | protein: 31.6g

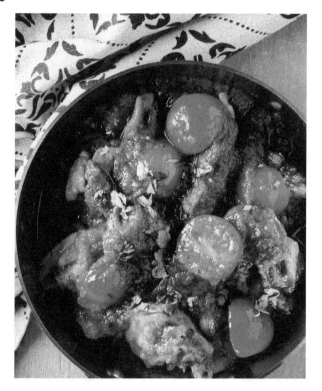

Ingredients:

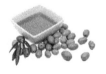

3 tablespoons olive oil, plus more for greasing the slow cooker

2½ pounds (1.1 kg) boneless lamb shoulder, cubed

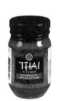

4 tablespoons curry paste

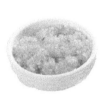

5 garlic cloves, finely chopped

2 onions, roughly chopped

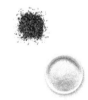

Salt and freshly ground black pepper, to taste

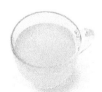

1 lamb stock cube

2 tomatoes, chopped

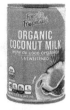

2½ cups unsweetened coconut milk

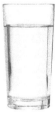

1 cup water

Fresh coriander, roughly chopped, for garnish

Full-fat Greek yogurt, to serve

GARLICKY LAMB LEG WITH ROSEMARY

Macros: Fat 40% | Protein 56% | Carbs 4%

Prep time: 15 minutes | Cook time: 30 minutes | Serves 8

1. Warm the olive oil in a nonstick skillet over medium-high heat.
2. Add lamb leg to the skillet, and sprinkle with salt and black pepper. Sear for 3 minutes until browned on both sides.
3. Remove the lamb leg from the skillet to a platter. Allow to cool for a few minutes, then rub with rosemary and garlic.
4. Pour the water into a pressure cooker with a steamer, then arrange the lamb leg on the steamer.
5. Put the pressure cooker lid on and cook for 30 minutes.
6. Release the pressure, and remove the lamb leg from the pressure cooker. Allow to cool for 10 minutes and slice to serve.

TIP: If you think the taste of this recipe is a little plain, you can try to top the lamb leg with your secret glaze or homemade sauce to gift more flavor to the lamb leg.

PER SERVING
calories: 366 | total fat: 16.2g | total carbs: 1.2g | fiber: 0.6g | net carbs: 0.6g | protein: 51.1g

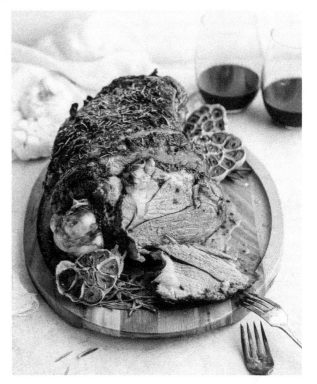

Ingredients:

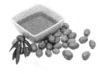

| 3 tablespoons extra-virgin olive oil | 4 pounds (1.8 kg) boneless leg of lamb | Salt and freshly ground black pepper, to taste | 2 tablespoons chopped rosemary | 1 tablespoon garlic |

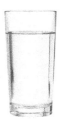

2 cups water

LAMB CHOPS WITH DRY RED WINE

Macros: Fat 79% | Protein 17% | Carbs 4%

Prep time: 10 minutes | Cook time: 40 minutes | Serves 4

1. Warm the olive oil in a nonstick skillet over medium-high heat.
2. Sauté the garlic and onion in the skillet for 3 minutes or until the onion is translucent.
3. Arrange the lamb chops on a clean work surface and rub with mint, sage, salt, and black pepper on both sides.
4. Add the lamb chops in the skillet and cook for 6 minutes until lightly browned. Flip the chops halfway through. Set aside.
5. Pour the dry red wine and water in the skillet. Bring to a boil, then cook until it reduces to half.
6. Add the cooked lamb chops back to the skillet. Lower the heat, and simmer for 30 minutes.
7. Remove them from the skillet and serve hot.

TIP: If you think the taste of this recipe is a little plain, you can try to top the lamb chops with your secret glaze or homemade sauce to gift more flavor to the lamb chops.

PER SERVING
calories: 341 | total fat: 29.8g | carbs: 3.6g | protein: 14.6g

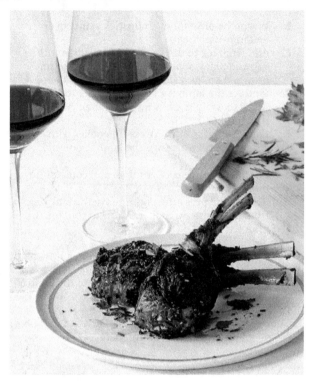

Ingredients:

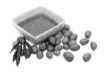

1 tablespoon olive oil

1 garlic clove, minced

½ onion, sliced

1 pound (454 g) lamb chops

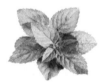

½ teaspoon mint

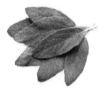

½ tablespoon sage

Salt and freshly ground black pepper, to taste

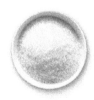

¼ cup dry red wine

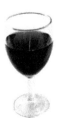

1 cup water

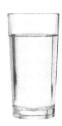

BANANA CREAMY FAT BOMBS

Macros: Fat 87% | Protein 10% | Carbs 3%

Prep time: 10 minutes | Cook time: 0 minutes | Serves 12 fat bombs

1. Line the 12-cup muffin tin with 12 paper liners.
2. Beat all the ingredients in a large bowl for 5 minutes until it has a thick and mousse-like consistency.
3. Pour the mixture into the 12 cups of the muffin tin. Put the muffin tin into the refrigerate to chill for 1 hour.
4. Remove the muffin tin from the refrigerator and serve chilled.

TIP: Store them in an airtight container in the refrigerator for up to 4 days, or more than 2 weeks in the freezer.

PER SERVING
calories: 125 | total fat: 12.1g | carbs: 0.9g | protein: 3.1g

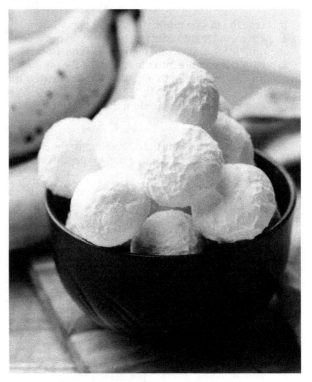

Ingredients:

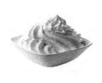
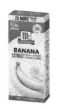

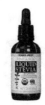

| ¾ cup heavy whipping cream | 1 tablespoon banana extract | 1¼ cups cream cheese, room temperature | 6 drops liquid stevia |

SPECIAL EQUIPMENT:

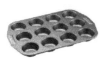

A 12-cup muffin tin

FROZEN BLUEBERRY KETO FAT BOMBS

Macros: Fat 92% | Protein 4% | Carbs 4%

Prep time: 10 minutes | Cook time: 0 minutes | Serves 12 fat bombs

1. Line the 12-cup muffin tin with 12 paper liners.
2. Put all the ingredients in a blender and process until it has a thick and mousse-like consistency.
3. Pour the mixture into the 12 cups of the muffin tin. Put the muffin tin into the refrigerate to chill for 1 to 3 hours.
4. Remove the muffin tin from the refrigerator and serve chilled.

TIP: Store them in an airtight container in the refrigerator for up to 4 days, or more than 2 weeks in the freezer.

PER SERVING
calories: 118 | total fat: 12.1g | carbs: 1.1g | protein: 1.2g

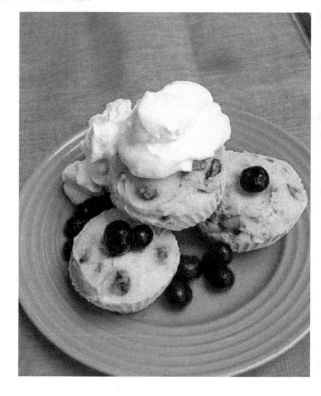

Ingredients:

½ cup blueberries, mashed

½ cup coconut oil, at room temperature

½ cup cream cheese, at room temperature

1 pinch nutmeg

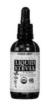

6 drops liquid stevia

SPECIAL EQUIPMENT:

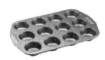

A 12-cup muffin tin

VANILLA AND CREAM CUSTARD

Macros: Fat 92% | Protein 4% | Carbs 4%

Prep time: 10 minutes | Cook time: 3 hours | Serves 4

1. Combine the beaten egg yolks, cream, vanilla extract, and stevia in a bowl, then pour them into a heat-proof dish.
2. Place the dish in the slow cooker. Pour the hot water into the slow cooker around the dish for about half way up the sides of the dish.
3. Put the slow cooker lid on and cook on HIGH for 3 hours.
4. Remove the custard from the slow cooker, and serve hot.

TIP: Store the custard in an airtight container in the refrigerator for no more than 3 days or it will lose its freshness.

PER SERVING
calories: 314 | total fat: 32.0g | carbs: 3.0g | protein: 3.0g

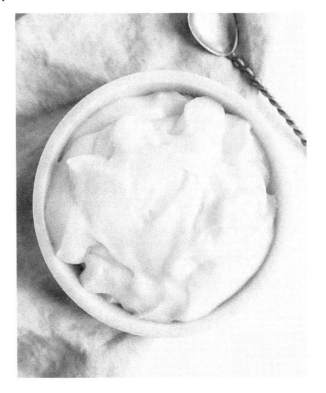

Ingredients:

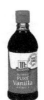
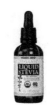

| 4 egg yolks, lightly beaten | 3 cups full-fat cream | 2 teaspoons vanilla extract | 5 drops of stevia |

STRAWBERRY CHEESECAKE

Macros: Fat 81% | Protein 10% | Carbs 9%

Prep time: 10 minutes | Cook time: 6 hours | Serves 8

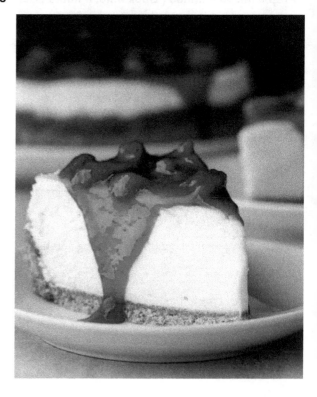

1. Make the base: Combine all the ingredients for the base in a bowl. Stir to mix well. Pour the mixture into a heat-proof dish.
2. Make the filling: Combine all the ingredients for the filling, except for the strawberries, in a blender. Process until creamy and smooth, then mix in the chopped strawberries.
3. Pour the strawberry mixture over the base mixture. Use a spoon to level the mixture.
4. Place the dish in the slow cooker. Pour the hot water into the slow cooker around the dish for about half way up the sides of the dish.
5. Put the slow cooker lid on and cook on LOW for 6 hours or until a knife inserted in the middle comes out clean.
6. Remove the dish from the slow cooker. Allow to cool for 10 minutes, then chill in the refrigerator for 1 hour before serving.

TIP: Store the cheesecake in an airtight container in the refrigerator for no more than 5 days or it will lose its freshness.

PER SERVING
calories: 421 | total fat: 38.7g | carbs: 9.7g | protein: 10.3g

BASE:

½ cup desiccated coconut

1 cup ground hazelnuts

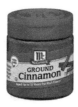

1 teaspoon ground cinnamon

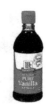

2 teaspoons vanilla extract

2 ounces (57 g) butter, melted

FILLING:

1 cup sour cream

2 cups cream cheese

2 eggs, lightly beaten

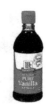

2 teaspoons vanilla extract

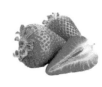

8 large strawberries, chopped

LEMONY CHEESECAKE

Macros: Fat 85% | Protein 8% | Carbs 7%

Prep time: 10 minutes | Cook time: 6 hours | Serves 10

1. Make the base: Combine all the ingredients for the base in a bowl. Stir to mix well. Pour the mixture into a heat-proof dish.
2. Make the filling: Combine all the ingredients for the filling in a blender. Process until creamy and smooth.
3. Pour the lemon mixture over the base mixture. Use a spoon to level the mixture.
4. Place the dish in the slow cooker. Pour the hot water into the slow cooker around the dish for about half way up the sides of the dish.
5. Put the slow cooker lid on and cook on LOW for 6 hours or until a knife inserted in the middle comes out clean.
6. Remove the dish from the slow cooker. Allow to cool for 10 minutes, then chill in the refrigerator for 1 hour. Spread the cream over the cheesecake before serving.

TIP: Store the cheesecake in an airtight container in the refrigerator for no more than 5 days or it will lose its freshness.

PER SERVING
calories: 351 | total fat: 34.3g | total carbs: 5.8g | fiber: 1.1g | net carbs: 4.7g | protein: 7.2g

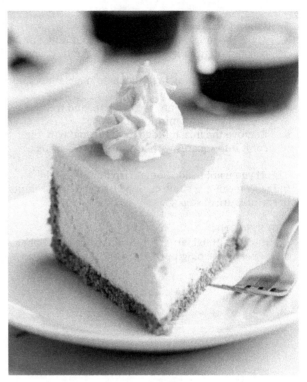

BASE:

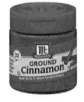

1 teaspoon cinnamon

1 cup pecans, finely ground

2 ounces (57 g) butter, melted

FILLING:

1 lemon

1 cup sour cream

2 cups cream cheese

2 eggs, lightly beaten

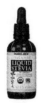

5 drops of stevia

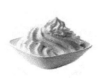

1 cup heavy whipping cream, for garnish

COCOA FUDGE

Macros: Fat 97% | Protein 1% | Carbs 2%

Prep time: 10 minutes | Cook time: 0 minutes | Serves 12 fudges

1. Line a loaf pan with parchment paper.
2. Make the fudge: Combine the coconut milk and coconut oil in a blender, then pulse until creamy and smooth.
3. Add the remaining ingredients to the blender and pulse to combine well.
4. Pour the mixture into the loaf pan, and freeze in the freezer for 15 minutes until set.
5. Remove the frozen fudge from the loaf pan, then cut it into squares with a knife before serving.

TIP: If you want to add some crisp flavor into the fudge, you can mix some crushed walnuts or hazelnuts in the mixture at step 3.

PER SERVING
calories: 173 | total fat: 20.1g | total carbs: 1.2g | fiber: 0.6g | net carbs: 0.6g | protein: 1.1g

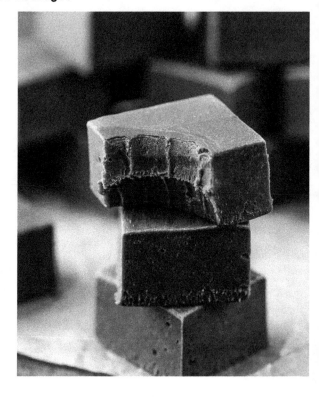

Ingredients:

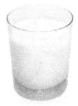

1 cup coconut oil, soft but still solid

¼ cup full-fat coconut milk

¼ cup organic cocoa powder

¼ cup Swerve confectioners style sweetener

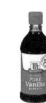

1 teaspoon vanilla oil or extract

½ teaspoon almond oil extract

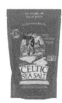

½ teaspoon Celtic sea salt

DESSERT

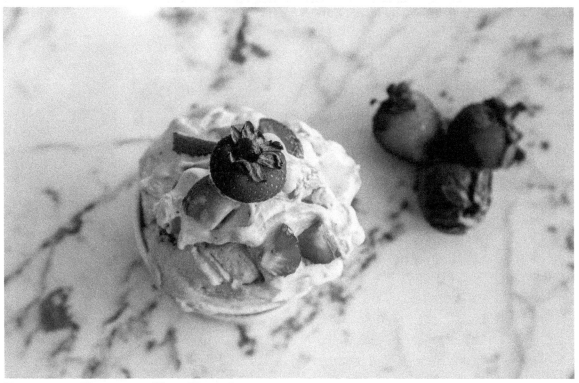

PEANUT BUTTER BLACKBERRY BARS

Macros: Fat 77% | Protein 14% | Carbs 9%

Prep time: 30 minutes | Cook time: 0 minutes | Serves 8 bars

1. Put all ingredients into a saucepan, and heat over medium-low heat until well combined. Stir constantly.
2. Pour the mixture into a blender, and process until the mixture is glossy.
3. Pour the mixture on a baking sheet lined with parchment paper.
4. Place the sheet in the freezer to chill for 30 minutes or until frozen.
5. Remove the frozen chunks from the freezer and cut into 8 bars before serving.

TIP: You can store the bars in an airtight container in the refrigerator for up to 4 days.

PER SERVING
calories: 252 | total fat: 21.5g | total carbs: 7.9g | fiber: 2.8g | net carbs: 5.1g | protein: 8.8g

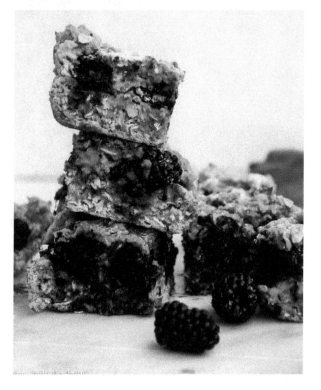

Ingredients:

1 cup peanut butter

½ cup coconut cream

½ cup blackberries (fresh or frozen)

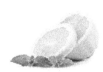

1 tablespoon lemon juice

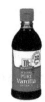

½ teaspoon vanilla extract

EASY BERRY BITES

Macros: Fat 98% | Protein 0% | Carbs 2%

Prep time: 35 minutes | Cook time: 0 minutes | Serves 6 bites

1. Melt the coconut oil in a saucepan over medium-low heat.
2. Pour the melted coconut oil into a blender, then add the berries and vanilla extract. Process until the mixture is glossy.
3. Pour the mixture on a baking sheet lined with parchment paper.
4. Place the sheet in the freezer to chill for 25 minutes or until frozen.
5. Remove the frozen chunks from the freezer and cut into 6 pieces before serving.

TIP: You can store the bites in an airtight container in the refrigerator for up to 4 days.

PER SERVING
calories: 342 | total fat: 37.4g | total carbs: 1.9g | fiber: 0.8g | net carbs: 1.1g | protein: 0g

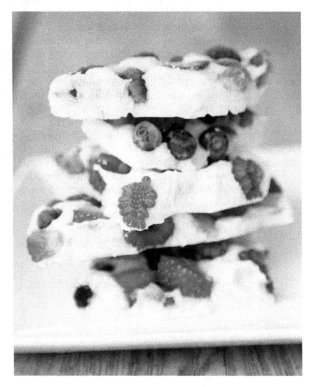

Ingredients:

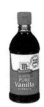

| 1 cup coconut oil | ½ cup mixed berries (fresh or frozen) | 1 teaspoon vanilla extract |

MATCHA BALLS WITH COCONUT

Macros: Fat 95% | Protein 1% | Carbs 4%

Prep time: 25 minutes | Cook time: 0 minutes | Serves 16 balls

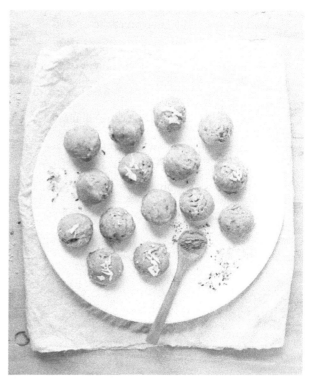

1. Combine all the ingredient, except for the shredded coconut, in a microwave-proof bowl. Microwave for 10 seconds until the coconut oil melts.
2. Stir the mixture in the bowl to combine well. Wrap the bowl in plastic and put it in the refrigerator to chill for 1 hour.
3. Spread half cup of shredded coconut on the bottom of a baking sheet lined with parchment paper.
4. Remove the bowl from the refrigerator and shape the frozen mixture into 16 balls with a tablespoon.
5. Roll the balls through the shredded coconut on the baking sheet, then top with remaining coconut.
6. Place the sheet in the refrigerator to chill for 15 more minutes.
7. Remove the balls from the refrigerator and serve chilled.

TIP: You can store the balls in an airtight container in the refrigerator for up to 12 days.

PER SERVING
calories: 263 | total fat: 27.8g | total carbs: 5.3g | fiber: 3.2g | net carbs: 2.1g | protein: 0.4g

Ingredients:

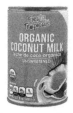

½ cup unsweetened coconut milk

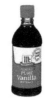

1 teaspoon vanilla extract

1 cup coconut butter

1 cup coconut oil

1½ teaspoons matcha green tea powder

2 tablespoons organic lemon zest

Sea salt, to taste

1 cup shredded coconut

EASY SESAME COOKIES

Macros: Fat 88% | Protein 6% | Carbs 6%

Prep time: 10 minutes | Cook time: 15 minutes | Serves 16 cookies

1. Preheat the oven to 375°F (190°C).
2. Combine all the dry ingredients in a bowl. Whisk together all the wet ingredients in a separate bowl.
3. Pour the wet mixture into the bowl for the dry ingredients. Stir until the mixture has a thick consistency and forms a dough.
4. Put the sesame seeds in a third bowl. Divide and shape the dough into 16 1½-inch balls, then dunk the balls in the bowl of sesame seeds to coat well.
5. Bash the balls until they are ½ inch thick, then put them on a baking sheet lined with parchment paper. Keep a little space between each of them.
6. Bake in the preheated oven for 15 minutes or until set and well browned.
7. Remove the cookies from the oven and allow to cool for a few minutes before serving.

TIP: You can store the cookies in an airtight container in the refrigerator for up to 5 days, or in the freezer for 1 month.

PER SERVING
calories: 174 | total fat: 17.2g | total carbs: 1.9g | fiber: 1.1g | net carbs: 0.8g | protein: 3.1g

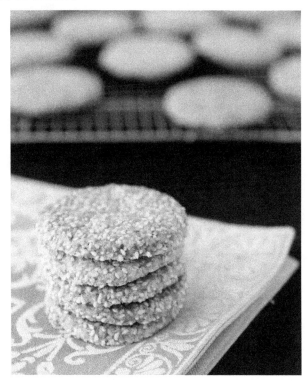

FRY:

⅓ cup monk fruit sweetener, granulated

¾ teaspoon baking powder

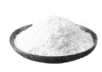

1 cup almond flour

WET:

1 egg

1 teaspoon toasted sesame oil

½ cup grass-fed butter, at room temperature

½ cup sesame seeds

MATCHA AND MACADAMIA BROWNIES

Macros: Fat 82% | Protein 12% | Carbs 6%

Prep time: 10 minutes | Cook time: 20 minutes | Serves 4

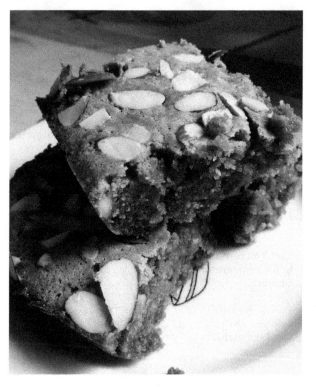

1. Preheat the oven to 350°F (180°C).
2. Combine the sweetener, melted butter, and salt in a bowl. Stir to mix well.
3. Separate the egg into the bowl, whisk to combine well.
4. Fold in the matcha powder, coconut flour, and baking powder, then add the macadamia nuts. Stir to combine.
5. Pour the mixture on a baking sheet lined with parchment paper. Level the mixture with a spoon to make sure it coat the bottom of the sheet evenly.
6. Cook in the preheated oven for 18 minutes or until a sharp knife inserted in the center of the brownies comes out clean.
7. Remove the brownies from the oven and slice to serve.

TIP: If you don't like the flavor of the macadamia nuts, you can replace it to walnuts or hazelnuts.

PER SERVING
calories: 244 | total fat: 22.1g | carbs: 4.2g | protein: 7.3g

Ingredients:

4 tablespoons Swerve confectioners style sweetener

¼ cup unsalted butter, melted

Salt, to taste

1 egg

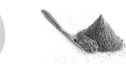

1 tablespoon tea matcha powder

¼ cup coconut flour

½ teaspoon baking powder

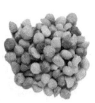

½ cup chopped macadamia nuts

POULTRY

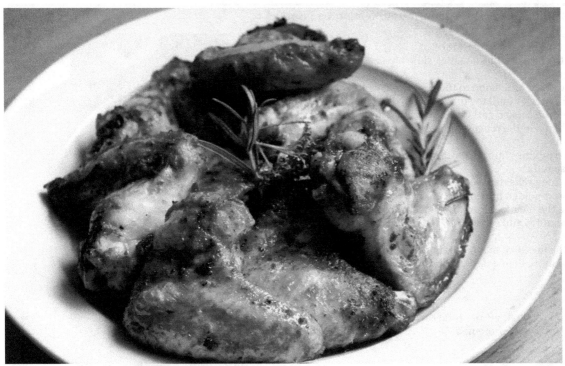

TURKEY MEATLOAF

Macros: Fat 70% | Protein 24% | Carbs 6%

Prep time: 10 minutes | Cook time: 1 hour 5 minutes | Serves 6

1. Preheat the oven to 350°F (180°C).
2. Warm the olive oil in a nonstick skillet over medium-high heat.
3. Add the garlic and onion to the skillet and sauté for 3 minutes or until the onion is translucent.
4. Transfer the cooked garlic and onion to a large bowl, then add the remaining ingredients. Stir to mix well.
5. Pour the mixture into a meatloaf pan, and press with a spatula.
6. Bake in the preheated oven for 1 hour until the meatloaf is golden brown.
7. Remove the meatloaf from the oven. Allow to cool for 10 minutes and serve.

TIP: Store the meatloaf in an airtight container in the fridge for no more than 4 days, or in the freezer for up to 3 months.

PER SERVING
calories: 356 | total fat: 28.1g | total carbs: 5.9g | fiber: 3.1g | net carbs: 2.8g | protein: 20.8g

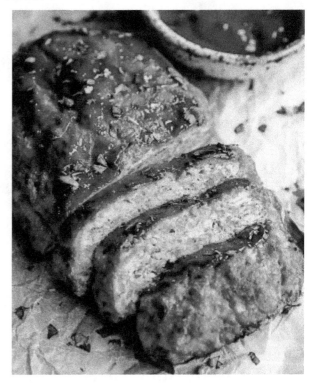

Ingredients:

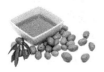

2 tablespoons extra-virgin olive oil

2 teaspoons minced garlic

½ onion, chopped

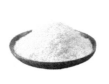

½ cup ground almonds

½ cup heavy whipping cream

1 large egg, beaten

1 pound ground turkey

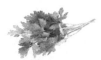

1 tablespoon chopped fresh parsley

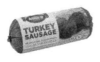

8 ounces (227 g) turkey sausage meat

Salt and freshly ground black pepper, to taste

TURKEY, BABY SPINACH, AND ZUCCHINI FRITTATA

Macros: Fat 70% | Protein 24% | Carbs 6%

Prep time: 15 minutes | Cook time: 30 minutes | Serves 4

1. Preheat the oven to 375°F (190°C).
2. Combine the beaten eggs and cream in a bowl. Sprinkle with salt and black pepper. Set aside until ready to use.
3. Warm the olive oil in an oven-safe skillet over medium-high heat.
4. Add the turkey breast to the skillet and cook for 6 to 8 minutes until an instant-read thermometer inserted in the thickest park of the turkey registers at least 150°F (66°C). Flip the turkey breast halfway through. Set aside.
5. Add the garlic and onion to the skillet and sauté for 3 minutes or until the onion is translucent.
6. Add the zucchini and spinach to the skillet and sauté for 4 minutes or until fork-tender.
7. Add the cooked turkey back to the skillet and stir to combine well.
8. Make the frittata: Pour the egg mixture over the turkey and cook for 3 minutes or until the eggs are set and no longer jiggle.
9. Place the oven-safe skillet in the preheated oven and bake for 20 minutes. Cut a small slit in the center, if raw eggs run into the cut, baking for another few minutes.

TIP: Store the frittata in an airtight container in the fridge for no more than 4 days, or in the freezer for up to 3 months.

PER SERVING
calories: 434 | total fat: 33.3g | total carbs: 6.7g | fiber: 2.1g | net carbs: 4.6g | protein: 27.1g

Ingredients:

6 large eggs, beaten

½ cup heavy whipping cream

Salt and freshly ground black pepper, to taste

3 tablespoons extra-virgin olive oil

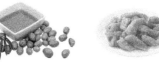

8 ounces (227 g) turkey breast, diced

½ onion, chopped

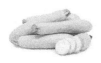

2 yellow zucchini, shredded

2 cups fresh baby spinach leaves

2 teaspoons garlic, minced

SPINACH AND OLIVE STUFFED CHICKEN WITH MOZZARELLA

Macros: Fat 53% | Protein 44% | Carbs 3%

Prep time: 10 minutes | Cook time: 4 hours | Serves 6

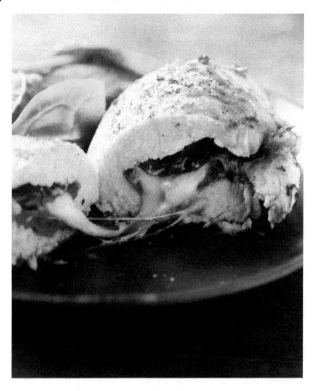

1. Cut through the chicken breasts horizontally, and leave the side of the chicken breast opposite to where you started intact.
2. Unfold the breasts like opening a book, and rub with olive oil, salt, and black pepper.
3. Arrange the spinach, olive, Mozzarella cheese, and garlic in the breasts, then fold.
4. Place the stuffed chicken breasts in the slow cooker, and top with tomatoes and dried mixed herbs.
5. Put the slow cooker lid on and cook on HIGH for 4 hours.
6. Scatter the extra Mozzarella cheese over the chicken breasts and put the slow cooker lid on, and cook until the cheese melts.
7. Remove the chicken from the slow cooker and serve hot.

TIP: To make this a complete meal, you can serve it with tomato and zucchini casserole, and dry red wine beef.

PER SERVING
calories: 492 | total fat: 29.3g | total carbs: 4.0g | fiber: 0.9g | net carbs: 3.1g | protein: 51.5g

Ingredients:

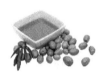

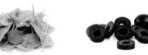

4 (6-ounce / 170-g) large chicken breasts, skin off

2 tablespoons extra-virgin olive oil

Salt and freshly ground black pepper, to taste

1 cup baby spinach, roughly chopped

12 black olives, pitted, chopped into chunks

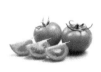

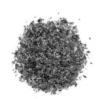

½ pound (227 g) sliced Mozzarella cheese, plus ½ cup for topping

4 garlic cloves, finely chopped

2 tomatoes, chopped

½ teaspoon dried mixed herbs

CHICKEN AND AVOCADO WRAPPED LETTUCE

Macros: Fat 72% | Protein 19% | Carbs 9%

Prep time: 10 minutes | Cook time: 5 minutes | Serves 4

1. Warm the olive oil in an oven-safe skillet over medium-high heat.
2. Put the chopped chicken breasts in the skillet, and sprinkle with salt and black pepper. Sauté for 5 minutes or until well browned. Set aside.
3. Combine the mashed avocado, thyme, mayo, and lemon juice in a bowl, then add the cooked chicken. Toss to mix well.
4. Divide and arrange the mixture on the lettuce leaves, then top with walnuts before serving.

TIP: To make this a complete meal, you can serve it with tomato and zucchini casserole, and dry red wine beef.

PER SERVING
calories: 253 | total fat: 20.1g | carbs: 5.9g | protein: 12.1g

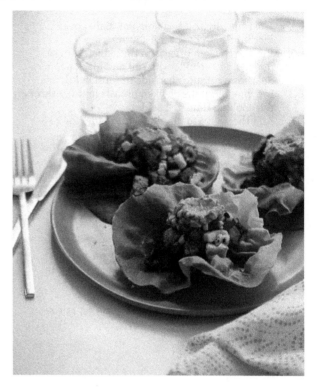

Ingredients:

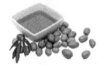

2 tablespoons extra-virgin olive oil

6 ounces (170 g) chicken breasts, chopped

¼ cup walnuts, chopped

½ avocado, peeled, pitted, and mashed

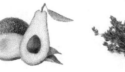

2 teaspoons thyme, fresh and chopped

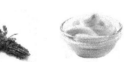

⅓ cup creamy mayonnaise, keto-friendly

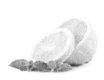

1 teaspoon freshly squeezed lemon juice

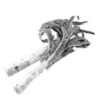

8 large lettuce leaves

Salt and freshly ground black pepper, to taste

SPICY CHICKEN BREASTS

Macros: Fat 69% | Protein 26% | Carbs 5%

Prep time: 10 minutes | Cook time: 25 minutes | Serves 4

1. Heat the olive oil in a nonstick skillet over medium-high heat until shimmering.
2. Put the chicken breasts in the skillet, skin side down, and sprinkle with salt and black pepper. Sear for 5 minutes per side or until lightly browned. Flip the chicken breasts halfway through the cooking time. Set aside.
3. Add the onion to the skillet and sauté for 4 minutes or until translucent.
4. Mix in the cream and paprika, then bring the mixture to a simmer.
5. Put the chicken back to the skillet, and simmer for an additional 5 minutes.
6. Remove the chicken breasts from the skillet. Spread the sour cream and parsley on top before serving.

TIP: To make this a complete meal, you can serve it with ratatouille, and rich crab and avocado broth.

PER SERVING
calories: 392 | total fat: 30.1g | carbs: 3.8g | protein: 25.1g

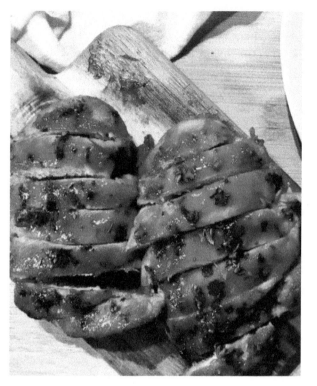

Ingredients:

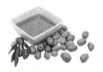

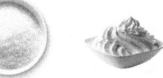

2 tablespoons olive oil

4 chicken breasts, skin on

Salt and freshly ground black pepper, to taste

½ cup heavy whipping cream

2 teaspoons smoked paprika

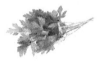

2 cups sour cream

2 tablespoons parsley, chopped

½ cup sweet onion, chopped

CHICKEN CAPRESE

Macros: Fat 65% | Protein 28% | Carbs 7%

Prep time: 15 minutes | Cook time: 40 minutes | Serves 4

1. Preheat the oven to 400°F (205°C).
2. Heat 2 tablespoons of the olive oil in an oven-safe skillet over medium-high heat until shimmering.
3. Put the chicken breasts in the skillet, and sprinkle with salt and black pepper. Sear for 5 minutes per side or until lightly browned. Flip the chicken breasts halfway through the cooking time. Set aside.
4. Make the sauce: Heat the remaining olive oil in the skillet over medium-high heat. Sauté the garlic in the skillet for 2 minutes until fragrant, then mix in the tomatoes, red pepper flakes, and basil. Sauté for another 5 minutes until well combined and has a thick consistency.
5. Put the chicken breasts back to the skillet, and spoon the sauce over to coat, then scatter the Mozzarella cheese over.
6. Put the skillet lid on and bake in the preheated oven for 25 minutes or until an instant-read thermometer inserted in the thickest part of the chicken breasts registers at least 165°F (74°C).
7. Remove the chicken breasts and sauce from the oven and serve hot.

TIP: To make this a complete meal, you can serve it with ratatouille, and rich crab and avocado broth.

PER SERVING
calories: 433 | total fat: 32.2g | total carbs: 8.9g | fiber: 3.1g | net carbs: 5.8g | protein: 29.1g

Ingredients:

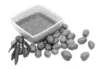

¼ cup extra-virgin olive oil, divided

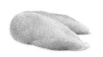

4 (4-ounce / 113-g) boneless chicken breasts

Salt and freshly ground black pepper, to taste

1 (28-ounce / 794-g) can diced tomatoes

Red pepper flakes, to taste

2 tablespoons chopped fresh basil

4 ounces (113 g) shredded Mozzarella cheese

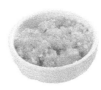

1 tablespoon minced garlic

RICOTTA, PROSCIUTTO, AND SPINACH CHICKEN ROLLATINI

Macros: Fat 64% | Protein 34% | Carbs 2%

Prep time: 15 minutes | Cook time: 35 minutes | Serves 4

1. Preheat the oven to 400°F (205°C).
2. Make the rollatini: On a clean work surface, put 1 ounce (28 g) of ricotta cheese on the center of a chicken breast, then top the ricotta cheese with a slice of prosciutto, and ¼ cup of the spinach. Repeat with the remaining chicken breasts, ricotta cheese, prosciutto, and spinach.
3. Roll up the chicken breasts to wrap the filling, then secure with two toothpicks. Set aside.
4. Whisk the eggs in a bowl. Combine the almond flour and Parmesan cheese in another bowl.
5. Dredge the chicken rollatini in the whisked eggs, then dunk in the almond flour mixture to coat well.
6. Heat the olive oil in an oven-safe skillet over medium heat until shimmering.
7. Arrange the chicken rollatini in the skillet, seam side down, and sprinkle with salt and black pepper. Fry for 10 minutes or until well browned. Gently flip them halfway through the cooking time.
8. Bake the chicken rollatini in the preheated oven for 25 minutes or until an instant-read thermometer inserted in the thickest part of the chicken breasts registers at least 165°F (74°C).
9. Transfer the chicken rollatini onto four plates. Remove the toothpicks and serve warm.

TIP: You can replace the chicken to eggplant slices as the wrapper, and omit the prosciutto to change this recipe into a vegetable recipe.

PER SERVING
calories: 439 | total fat: 30.1g | total carbs: 1.9g | fiber: 0g | net carbs: 1.9g | protein: 40.2g

Ingredients:

4 ounces (113 g) ricotta cheese

4 (3-ounce / 85-g) boneless skinless chicken breasts, pounded to about ⅓-inch thick

4 (1-ounce / 28-g) slices prosciutto

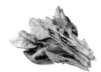

1 cup fresh spinach

2 eggs

SPECIAL EQUIPMENT:

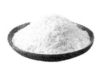

½ cup almond flour

½ cup grated Parmesan cheese

¼ cup extra-virgin olive oil

Salt and freshly ground black pepper, to taste

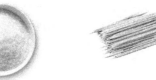

8 toothpicks, soak in water for at least 30 minutes

SPICY SAUSAGE AND CHICKEN SCARPARIELLO

Macros: Fat 74% | Protein 22% | Carbs 4%

Prep time: 10 minutes | Cook time: 45 minutes | Serves 6

1. Preheat the oven to 425°F (220°C).
2. Heat 2 tablespoons of the olive oil in an oven-safe skillet over medium-high heat until shimmering.
3. Put the sausage and chicken thighs in the skillet, and sprinkle with salt and black pepper. Sear for 5 minutes per side or until lightly browned. Flip the them halfway through the cooking time. Set aside.
4. Arrange the skillet in the preheated oven and bake for 25 minutes or until an instant-read thermometer inserted in the thickest part of the chicken breasts registers at least 165°F (74°C). Transfer them into a plate. Set aside.
5. Heat the remaining olive oil in the skillet over medium-high heat until shimmering.
6. Sauté the pimiento and garlic in the skillet for 3 minutes until fragrant, then pour the dry white wine over for deglazing.
7. Pour the chicken stock in the skillet, then bring them to a boil.Turn down the heat to low and simmer for 6 minutes until it reduces to half.
8. Put the sausage and chicken back to the skillet, and toss to coat well. Transfer them to a plate, and spread the parsley on top before serving.

TIP: To make this a complete meal, you can serve it with sautéed zucchini, or creamed spinach.

PER SERVING
calories: 372 | total fat: 30.1g | total carbs: 2.9g | fiber: 0g | net carbs: 2.9g | protein: 19.1g

Ingredients:

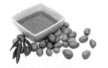

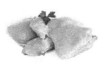

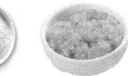

| 3 tablespoons extra-virgin olive oil, divided | ½ pound (227 g) Italian sausage (sweet or hot) | 1 pound (454 g) boneless chicken thighs | Salt and freshly ground black pepper, to taste | 1 tablespoon minced garlic |

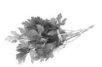

| ¼ cup dry white wine | 1 cup chicken stock | 2 tablespoons chopped fresh parsley | 1 pimiento, chopped |

CHICKEN THIGH AND TOMATO BRAISE

Macros: Fat 70% | Protein 20% | Carbs 10%

Prep time: 10 minutes | Cook time: 4 hours | Serves 4

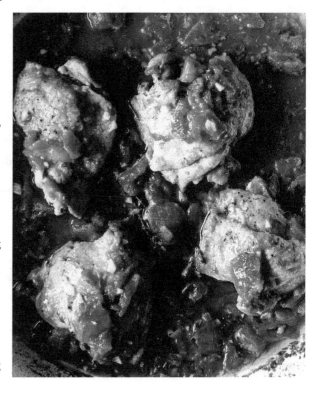

1. Coat the insert of the slow cooker with 1 tablespoon olive oil.
2. Heat the remaining olive oil in a nonstick skillet over medium-high heat, then put the chicken thighs in the skillet and sprinkle salt and black pepper to season.
3. Sear the chicken thighs for 10 minutes or until well browned. Flip them halfway through the cooking time.
4. Put the chicken thighs, stock, tomatoes, oregano, garlic, and red pepper flakes into the slow cooker. Stir to coat the chicken thighs well.
5. Put the slow cooker lid on and cook on HIGH for 4 hours until an instant-read thermometer inserted in the thickest part of the chicken thighs registers at least 165°F (74°C).
6. Transfer the chicken thighs to four plates. Pour the sauce which remains in the slow cooker over the chicken thighs and top with fresh parsley before serving warm.

TIP: To cook this dish with a faster way: Preheat the oven to 375°F (190°C). Toss all the ingredients in a baking pan, then cover with aluminum foil. Cook in the preheated oven for 1 hour and 30 minutes.

PER SERVING
calories: 469 | total fat: 36.1g | total carbs: 13.7g | fiber: 7.3g | net carbs: 6.4g | protein: 24.2g

Ingredients:

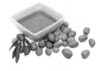
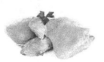

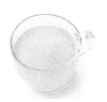
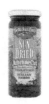
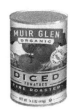

¼ cup olive oil, divided

4 (4-ounce / 113-g) boneless chicken thighs

Salt and freshly ground black pepper, to taste

½ cup chicken stock

4 ounces (113 g) julienned oil-packed sun-dried tomatoes

1 (28-ounce / 794-g) can sodium-free diced tomatoes

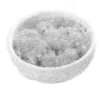

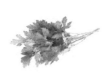

2 tablespoons dried oregano

2 tablespoons minced garlic

Red pepper flakes, to taste

2 tablespoons chopped fresh parsley

BRAISED CHICKEN, BACON, AND MUSHROOMS

Macros: Fat 71% | Protein 22% | Carbs 7%

Prep time: 15 minutes | Cook time: 7 hours | Serves 8

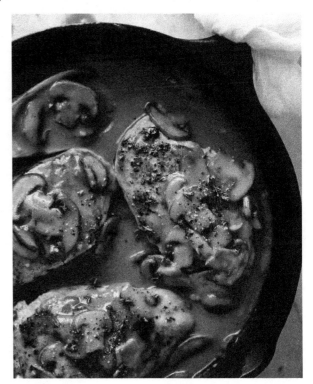

1. Coat the insert of the slow cooker with 1 tablespoon coconut oil.
2. Heat the remaining coconut oil in a nonstick skillet over medium-high heat, then put the bacon in the skillet and cook for 5 minutes or until curls and buckle. Flip the bacon halfway through the cooking time. Set aside.
3. Put the chicken drumsticks in the skillet and cook for 5 minutes or until well browned. Flip the drumsticks halfway through the cooking time.
4. Transfer the chicken drumsticks and cooked bacon into the slow cooker, then add the mushrooms, broth, garlic, thyme, and onion. Stir to mix well.
5. Cover the slow cooker lid on and cook on LOW for 7 hours.
6. Remove them from the slow cooker and top with coconut cream before serving.

TIP: To make this a complete meal, you can serve it with creamy asparagus and seafood soup.

PER SERVING
calories: 408 | total fat: 34.2g | total carbs: 4.9g | fiber: 2.1g | net carbs: 2.8g | protein: 22.1g

Ingredients:

3 tablespoons coconut oil, divided

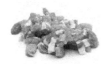

¼ pound (113 g) bacon, diced

2 pounds (907 g) chicken drumsticks

2 cups quartered button mushrooms

½ cup chicken broth

1 tablespoon garlic, minced

2 teaspoons thyme, chopped

1 sweet onion, diced

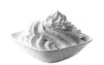

1 cup coconut cream

AROMATIC ROASTED DUCK

Macros: Fat 69% | Protein 29% | Carbs 2%

Prep time: 15 minutes | Cook time: 7 hours | Serves 8

1. Coat the insert of the slow cooker with 1 tablespoon olive oil.
2. Brush the whole duck with the remaining olive oil on all sides, and sprinkle salt and black pepper to season.
3. Stuff the cavity of the duck with cinnamon, thyme, and garlic.
4. Spread the chopped onion on the bottom of the insert of the slow cooker, then put the duck in the slow cooker. Pour the chicken broth over.
5. Cover the slow cooker lid on and cook on LOW for 7 hours or until an instant-read thermometer inserted in the center of the duck registers at least 180°F (82°C).
6. Remove the duck from the oven to a large plate, and paste with the sauce remains in the slow cooker. Remove the cinnamon stick and thyme sprigs from the duck and slice to serve.

TIP: To make this a complete meal, you can serve it with creamy asparagus and seafood soup.

PER SERVING
calories: 367 | total fat: 28.3g | total carbs: 1.8g | fiber: 1.0g | net carbs: 0.8g | protein: 28.7g

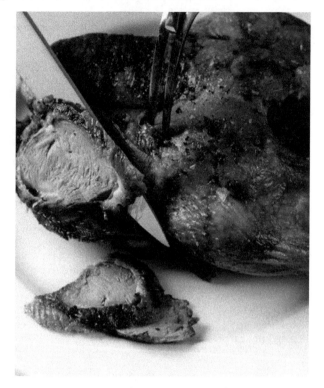

Ingredients:

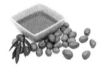

3 tablespoons extra-virgin olive oil, divided

1 (2½-pound / 1.1-kg) whole duck, giblets removed

Salt and freshly ground black pepper, to taste

6 thyme sprigs, chopped

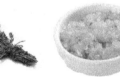

4 garlic cloves, crushed

1 sweet onion, coarsely chopped

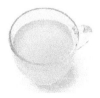

¼ cup chicken broth

1 cinnamon stick, broken into several pieces

TOMATO AND EGGPLANT WITH RICH CHICKEN THIGHS

Macros: Fat 76% | Protein 22% | Carbs 2%

Prep time: 10 minutes | Cook time: 20 minutes | Serves 4

1. Put the butter in a nonstick skillet, melt over medium heat.
2. Put the chicken thighs in the skillet, and sprinkle with salt and black pepper. Fry for 8 minutes or until well browned. Flip the chicken thighs halfway through the cooking time.
3. Transfer the chicken thighs to a plate, then add the garlic to the skillet. Sauté in the remaining butter for 2 minutes or until fragrant.
4. Add the tomatoes to the skillet and sauté for 8 minutes or until lightly softened.
5. Add the eggplant and basil to the skillet, and cook for 4 more minutes until tender. Sprinkle salt and black pepper to season.
6. Put the chicken thighs back to the skillet, and spoon the sauce in the skillet over the chicken thighs to coat well.
7. Put the lid on and simmer for 3 minutes or until the internal temperature of the chicken thighs reach at least 165°F (74°C).
8. Transfer the chicken and the sauce to a large plate and serve with more basil on top.

TIP: To make this a complete meal, you can serve it with mashed cauliflower and jambalaya broth.

PER SERVING
calories: 469 | total fat: 39.7g | carbs: 1.9g | protein: 26.1g

Ingredients:

2 tablespoons butter

1 pound (454 g) chicken thighs

Salt and freshly ground black pepper, to taste

1 (14-ounce / 397-g) can whole tomatoes

1 eggplant, diced

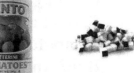

10 fresh basil leaves, chopped, plus more for garnish

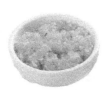

2 cloves garlic, minced

SOUP AND STEW

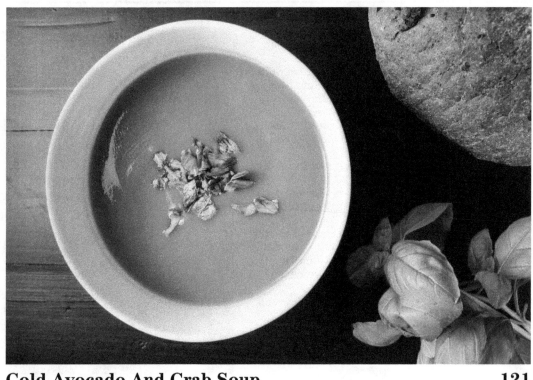

COLD AVOCADO AND CRAB SOUP

Macros: Fat 70% | Protein 23% | Carbs 7%

Prep time: 15 minutes | Cook time: 0 minutes | Serves 6

1. Combine all the ingredients, except for the crab meat, in a blender. Process until smooth.
2. Pour the soup in a large bowl. Add the crab meat into the soup and serve immediately

TIP: To make this a complete meal, you can serve it with shrimp skewers and garlicky roasted broccoli.

PER SERVING
calories: 298 | total fat: 23.1g | total carbs: 8.5g | fiber: 4.1g | net carbs: 4.4g | protein: 17.1g

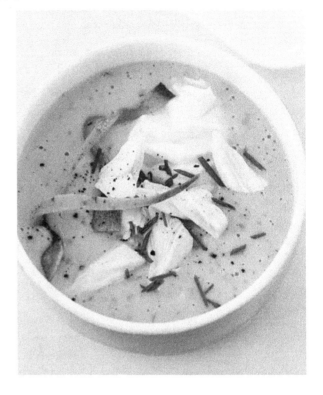

Ingredients:

½ onion, diced

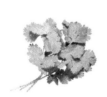

½ cup fresh cilantro, roughly chopped

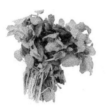

1 cup watercress

1 cup heavy whipping cream

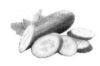

1 English cucumber, cut into chunks

2 avocados, diced

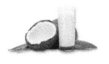

2 cups coconut water

2 teaspoons ground cumin

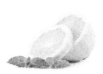

Juice of 1 lime

Salt and freshly ground black pepper, to taste

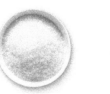

1 pound (454 g) cooked crab meat

SMOKED SALMON AND LEEK SOUP

Macros: Fat 72% | Protein 19% | Carbs 9%

Prep time: 10 minutes | Cook time: 3 hours | Serves 6

1. Coat the insert of the slow cooker with 2 tablespoons olive oil.
2. Combine the salmon, stock cube, leek, garlic, onion, salt, and water in the slow cooker. Stir to mix well.
3. Put the slow cooker lid on and cook on LOW for 2 hours, then mix in the cream and cook for an additional 1 hour.
4. Remove the soup from the slow cooker to a large bowl. Serve warm.

TIP: To make this a complete meal, you can add a touch of cracked pepper and serve it with shrimp skewers and garlicky roasted asparagus.

PER SERVING
calories: 219 | total fat: 17.9g | total carbs: 5.0g | fiber: 0.5g | net carbs: 4.5g | protein: 10.0g

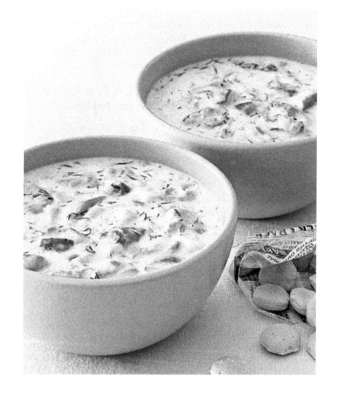

Ingredients:

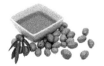

2 tablespoons extra-virgin olive oil

½ pound (227 g) smoked salmon, roughly chopped

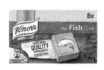

1 fish stock cube

1 leek, finely chopped

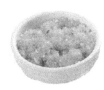

4 garlic cloves, crushed

1 small onion, finely chopped

Salt, to taste

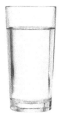

1 cup water

2 cups heavy whipping cream

SPICY AND SOUR CHICKEN STEW

Macros: Fat 65% | Protein 31% | Carbs 4%

Prep time: 10 minutes | Cook time: 6 hours | Serves 6

1. Coat the insert of the slow cooker with 2 tablespoons olive oil.
2. Combine the remaining ingredients, except for the coriander, in the slow cooker. Stir to mix well.
3. Put the slow cooker lid on and cook on LOW for 6 hours.
4. Transfer the stew to a large bowl. Top it with coriander and slice to serve.

TIP: To make this a complete meal, you can top the stew with avocado slices and serve it with Parmesan stuffed zucchini roast.

PER SERVING
calories: 445 | total fat: 32.2g | total carbs: 4.9g | fiber: 1.1g | net carbs: 3.8g | protein: 32.6g

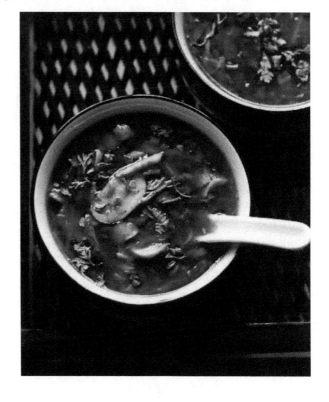

Ingredients:

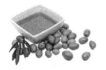

2 tablespoons extra-virgin olive oil

6 chicken thighs, skin on, boneless

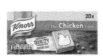

1 chicken stock cube

1 red chili, finely chopped

1 small onion, finely chopped

2 limes

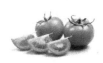

2 tins chopped tomatoes

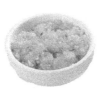

3 garlic cloves, crushed

Salt and freshly ground black pepper, to taste

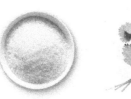

Large handful of fresh coriander, chopped

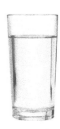

1 cup water

LAMB CURRY STEW

Macros: Fat 40% | Protein 53% | Carbs 7%

Prep time: 15 minutes | Cook time: 50 minutes | Serves 4

1. Heat the olive oil in a nonstick skillet over medium-high heat until shimmering.
2. Add the onion to the skillet and sauté for 4 minutes or until translucent.
3. Add the remaining ingredients and sauté to combine well.
4. Transfer all of them into a pressure cooker. Put the lid on and cook for 50 minutes.
5. Release the pressure, then remove the stew from the pressure cooker to a large bowl and serve warm.

TIP: To make this a complete meal, you can serve it with arugula and fennel salad with lemon vinaigrette, or dry red wine beef steak.

PER SERVING
calories: 386 | total fat: 17.1g | total carbs: 5.3g | fiber: 2.1g | net carbs: 3.2g | protein: 50.9g

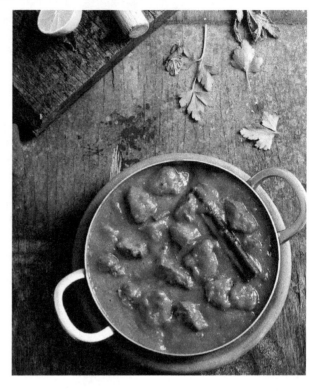

Ingredients:

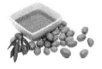

1 tablespoon olive oil

1 small yellow onion, chopped

1½ pounds (680 g) boneless lamb shoulder, chopped

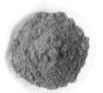

1 tablespoon curry powder

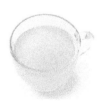

1½ cups chicken broth

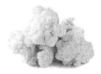

2 cups chopped cauliflower

Salt and freshly ground black pepper, to taste

CREAMY CHICKEN POT PIE SOUP

Macros: Fat 70% | Protein 25% | Carbs 5%

Prep time: 20 minutes | Cook time: 35 minutes | Serves 6

1. Heat the olive oil in a stockpot over medium-high heat until shimmering.
2. Add the chicken chunks to the pot and sauté for 10 minutes or until well browned. Transfer the chicken to a plate. Set aside until ready to use.
3. Heat the remaining olive oil in the stockpot over medium-high heat.
4. Add the mushrooms, celery, onion, and garlic to the pot and sauté for 6 minutes or until fork-tender.
5. Pour the chicken broth over, then add the cooked chicken chunks to the pot. Stir to mix well, and bring the soup to a boil.
6. Turn down the heat to low, and simmer the for 15 minutes or until the vegetables are soft and the internal temperature of the chicken reaches at least 165°F (74°C).
7. Mix in the green beans, cream cheese, cream, thyme, salt, and black pepper, then simmer for 3 more minutes.
8. Remove the soup from the stockpot and serve hot.

TIP: To make this a complete meal, you can serve it with arugula and fennel salad with lemon vinaigrette, or pork patties.

PER SERVING
calories: 338 | total fat: 26.1g | total carbs: 6.8g | fiber: 2.2g | net carbs: 4.6g | protein: 20.1g

Ingredients:

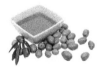

2 tablespoons extra-virgin olive oil, divided

1 pound (454 g) skinless chicken breast, cut into ½-inch chunks

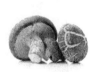

1 cup mushrooms, quartered

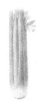

2 celery stalks, chopped

1 onion, chopped

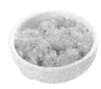

1 tablespoon garlic, minced

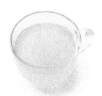

5 cups low-sodium chicken broth

1 cup green beans, chopped

¼ cup cream cheese

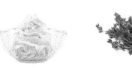

1 cup heavy whipping cream

1 tablespoon fresh thyme, chopped

Salt and freshly ground black pepper, to taste

SAUERKRAUT AND SAUSAGE SOUP

Macros: Fat 75% | Protein 18% | Carbs 7%

Prep time: 15 minutes | Cook time: 6 hours | Serves 6

1. Coat the insert of the slow cooker with olive oil.
2. Combine the remaining ingredients, except for the sour cream and parsley, in the slow cooker. Stir to mix well.
3. Put the slow cooker lid on and cook on LOW for 6 hours.
4. Transfer the soup into a large bowl, and mix in the sour cream. Top with parsley and serve warm.

TIP: Because the sauerkraut is high in sodium, so the salt is not necessary in the ingredients of this recipe.

PER SERVING
calories: 333 | total fat: 28.1g | total carbs: 5.8g | fiber: 2.1g | net carbs: 3.7g | protein: 15.1g

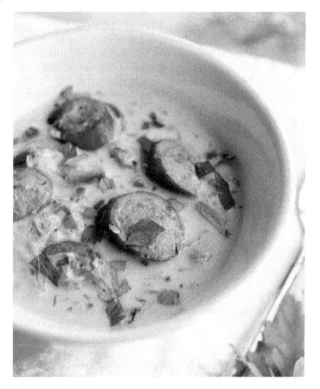

Ingredients:

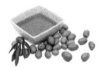

1 tablespoon extra-virgin olive oil

1 pound (454 g) organic sausage, cooked and sliced

2 cups sauerkraut

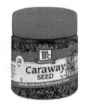

½ teaspoon caraway seeds

1 sweet onion, chopped

1 tablespoon hot mustard

2 tablespoons butter

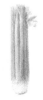

2 celery stalks, chopped

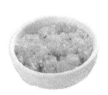

2 teaspoons minced garlic

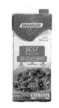

6 cups beef broth

½ cup sour cream

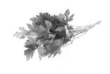

2 tablespoons chopped fresh parsley, for garnish

JAMBALAYA BROTH

Macros: Fat 70% | Protein 25% | Carbs 5%

Prep time: 15 minutes | Cook time: 6 hours 30 minutes | Serves 8

1. Coat the insert of the slow cooker with olive oil.
2. Combine the chicken, sausage, broth, tomatoes, onion, jalapeño, bell pepper, Cajun seasoning, and garlic in the slow cooker. Stir to mix well.
3. Put the slow cooker lid on and cook on LOW for 6 hours.
4. Add the shrimp and cook for an additional 30 minutes or until the fresh of the shrimp is opaque and a little white in color.
5. Transfer the soup into a large bowl. Add the avocado, sour cream, and cilantro, then stir to mix well before serving warm.

TIP: To make this a complete meal, you can serve it with spinach salad and jerk pork.

PER SERVING
calories: 402 | total fat: 31.1g | total carbs: 8.9g | fiber: 4.2g | net carbs: 4.7g | protein: 24.2g

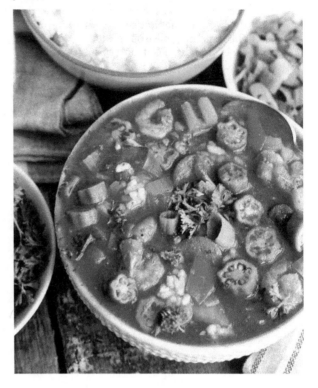

Ingredients:

| 1 tablespoon extra-virgin olive oil | 6 cups chicken broth | 1 (28-ounce / 794-g) can tomatoes, diced | 1 pound (454 g) spicy organic sausage, sliced | 1 cup cooked chicken, chopped | 1 red bell pepper, chopped | ½ sweet onion, chopped |

| 1 jalapeño pepper, chopped | 2 teaspoons garlic, minced | 3 tablespoons Cajun seasoning | ½ pound (227 g) medium shrimp, peeled, deveined, and chopped | ½ cup sour cream, for garnish | 1 avocado, diced, for garnish | 2 tablespoons chopped cilantro, for garnish |

BEEF AND PUMPKIN STEW

Macros: Fat 67% | Protein 25% | Carbs 8%

Prep time: 15 minutes | Cook time: 8 hours | Serves 6

1. Coat the insert of the slow cooker with olive oil.
2. Heat the remaining olive oil in a nonstick skillet. Add the beef to the skillet, and sprinkle salt and pepper to season.
3. Cook the beef for 7 minutes or until well browned. Flip the beef halfway through the cooking time.
4. Put the cooked beef into the slow cooker, then add the remaining ingredients, except for the parsley, to the slow cooker. Stir to mix well.
5. Put the slow cooker lid on and cook on LOW for 8 hours or until the internal temperature of the beef reaches at least 145°F (63°C).
6. Remove the stew from the slow cooker and top with parsley before serving.

TIP: To make this a complete meal, you can serve it with buttered spinach salad and zucchini carbonara.

PER SERVING
calories: 462 | total fat: 34.1g | total carbs: 9.9g | fiber: 3.2g | net carbs: 6.7g | protein: 32.1g

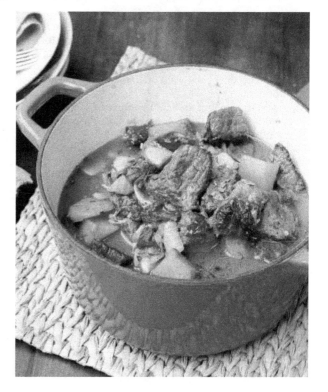

Ingredients:

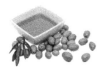

3 tablespoons extra-virgin olive oil, divided

1 (2-pound / 907-g) beef chuck roast, cut into 1-inch chunks

½ teaspoon salt

¼ teaspoon freshly ground black pepper

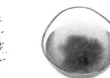

¼ cup apple cider vinegar

½ sweet onion, chopped

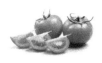

1 cup diced tomatoes

1 teaspoon dried thyme

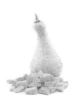

1½ cups pumpkin, cut into 1-inch chunks

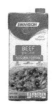

2 cups beef broth

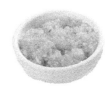

2 teaspoons minced garlic

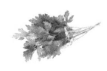

1 tablespoon chopped fresh parsley, for garnish

CAULIFLOWER AND CELERY SOUP WITH CRISP BACON

Macros: Fat 67% | Protein 25% | Carbs 8%

Prep time: 5 minutes | Cook time: 20 minutes | Serves 4

1. Heat the olive oil in a stockpot over medium heat until shimmering.
2. Add the onion to the pot and sauté for 3 minutes or until translucent.
3. Add the cauliflower florets and celery root to the pot and sauté for 3 minutes or until tender.
4. Pour the water into the pot, and sprinkle salt and black pepper to season. Stir to combine well and bring to a boil.
5. Turn down the heat to low and put the lid on to cook for 10 minutes.
6. Use an immersion blender to mix the ingredients in the soup entirely, then mix in the cheese and almond milk.
7. Fry the bacon in a nonstick skillet over high heat for 5 minutes or until curls and buckle. Flip the bacon halfway through the cooking time.
8. Divide the soup into four bowls and top with bacon. Serve hot.

TIP: To make this a complete meal, you can serve it with garlicky roasted broccoli and lettuce-wrapped chicken bites.

PER SERVING
calories: 365 | total fat: 27.2g | carbs: 7.4g | protein: 22.7g

Ingredients:

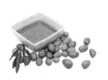

2 tablespoons olive oil

1 onion, chopped

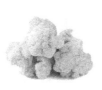

1 head cauliflower, cut into florets

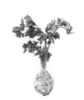

¼ celery root, grated

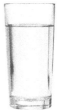

3 cups water

1 cup white Cheddar cheese, shredded

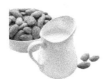

1 cup almond milk

2 ounces (57 g) bacon, cut into strips

Salt and freshly ground black pepper, to taste

SMOOTHY GREEN SOUP

Macros: Fat 81% | Protein 10% | Carbs 9%

Prep time: 5 minutes | Cook time: 25 minutes | Serves 4

1. Heat the coconut oil in a stockpot over medium heat until shimmering.
2. Add the leeks, onion, and garlic to the pot and cook for 5 minutes or until the onion is translucent.
3. Add the broccoli to the pot and cook for 5 minutes more or until tender.
4. Pour the vegetable stock in the pot, and add the bay leaf. Put the lid on and bring the soup to a boil.
5. Turn down the heat to low and simmer for 10 minutes.
6. Add the spinach to the pot and simmer for 3 minutes. Use an immersion blender to fully mix the soup. Mix in the the coconut milk, then season with salt and black pepper.
7. Discard the bay leaf and divide the soup into four bowls, then top with coconut yogurt before serving.

TIP: To make this a complete meal, you can serve it with roasted cauliflower and chicken meatloaf.

PER SERVING
calories: 273 | total fat: 24.6g | carbs: 4.1g | protein: 4.6g

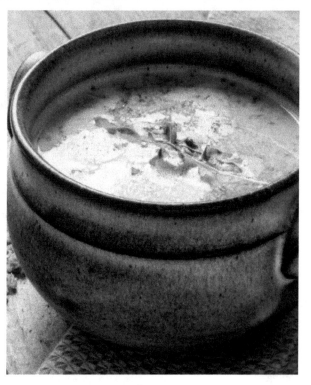

Ingredients:

2 tablespoons coconut oil

½ cup leeks

1 onion, chopped

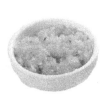

1 garlic clove, minced

1 broccoli head, chopped

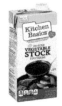

3 cups vegetable stock

1 bay leaf

1 cup spinach, blanched

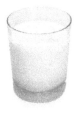

½ cup coconut milk

Salt and freshly ground black pepper, to taste

2 tablespoons coconut yogurt, for garnish

RICH CUCUMBER AND AVOCADO SOUP WITH TOMATO

Macros: Fat 81% | Protein 10% | Carbs 9%

Prep time: 10 minutes | Cook time: 0 minutes | Serves 4

1. Put the all the ingredients, except for the avocado and tomatoes, in a food processor. Process for 2 minutes or until it has a mousse-like consistency.
2. Transfer the soup into a large bowl, then spread the avocado and tomatoes on top.
3. Wrap the bowl in plastic and refrigerate for 2 hours before serving or serve immediately.

TIP: To make this a complete meal, you can serve it with fiery kale with garlic and braised chicken and mushrooms.

PER SERVING
calories: 344 | total fat: 26.2g | carbs: 5.1g | protein: 10.2g

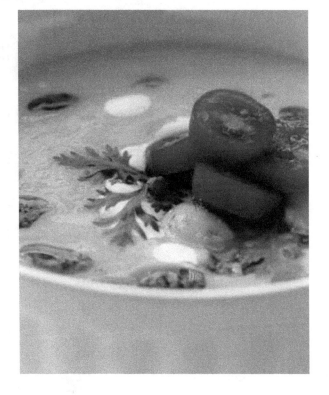

Ingredients:

½ cup plain Greek yogurt

1 garlic clove, minced

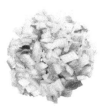

1 small onion, chopped

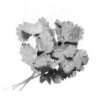

1 tablespoon cilantro, chopped

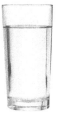

1½ cups water

2 limes, juiced

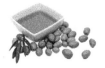

3 tablespoons olive oil

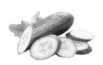

4 large cucumbers, chopped

Salt and freshly ground black pepper, to taste

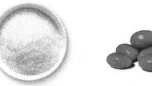

2 chopped tomatoes, for garnish

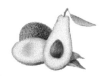

1 chopped avocado, for garnish

MEASUREMENT CONVERSION CHART

VOLUME EQUIVALENTS(DRY)

US STANDARD	METRIC (APPROXIMATE)
1/8 teaspoon	0.5 mL
1/4 teaspoon	1 mL
1/2 teaspoon	2 mL
3/4 teaspoon	4 mL
1 teaspoon	5 mL
1 tablespoon	15 mL
1/4 cup	59 mL
1/2 cup	118 mL
3/4 cup	177 mL
1 cup	235 mL
2 cups	475 mL
3 cups	700 mL
4 cups	1 L

VOLUME EQUIVALENTS(LIQUID)

US STANDARD	US STANDARD (OUNCES)	METRIC (APPROXIMATE)
2 tablespoons	1 fl.oz.	30 mL
1/4 cup	2 fl.oz.	60 mL
1/2 cup	4 fl.oz.	120 mL
1 cup	8 fl.oz.	240 mL
1 1/2 cup	12 fl.oz.	355 mL
2 cups or 1 pint	16 fl.oz.	475 mL
4 cups or 1 quart	32 fl.oz.	1 L
1 gallon	128 fl.oz.	4 L

TEMPERATURES EQUIVALENTS

FAHRENHEIT(F)	CELSIUS(C) (APPROXIMATE)
225 °F	107 °C
250 °F	120 °C
275 °F	135 °C
300 °F	150 °C
325 °F	160 °C
350 °F	180 °C
375 °F	190 °C
400 °F	205 °C
425 °F	220 °C
450 °F	235 °C
475 °F	245 °C
500 °F	260 °C

WEIGHT EQUIVALENTS

US STANDARD	METRIC (APPROXIMATE)
1 ounce	28 g
2 ounces	57 g
5 ounces	142 g
10 ounces	284 g
15 ounces	425 g
16 ounces (1 pound)	455 g
1.5 pounds	680 g
2 pounds	907 g

Dear Readers and Friends:

This is an invitation to step closer to us by voicing your opinion about our book. We are a group of dietitians and nutritionists who are so keen about diets, nutrition, and lifestyle that we have devoted our past 6 years researching, developing, testing, and writing recipes and cookbooks. This is the profession we take so much pride in, and we strive to write high-quality recipes and produce value-packed cookbooks. If you like our books, please do us a favor and leave an objective, honest and detailed review on our amazon page, the more specific, the better! It may take only a couple of minutes, but would mean the world to us. We will never stop devoting our careers and minds to producing more high-quality cookbooks to serve you better.

Additionally, You can get one book named keto diet mistakes for beginners as a free bonus from the link: https://mailchi.mp/0c3fd48025c3/keto-diet-cookbook, it would be appreciated if you like it.

CPSIA information can be obtained
at www.ICGtesting.com
Printed in the USA
LVHW062000220920
666814LV00003B/48